COMPACT *Research*

Diet Drugs

Drugs

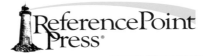

ReferencePoint Press®

San Diego, CA

Other books in the Compact Research Drugs set:

Antidepressants
Bath Salts and Other Synthetic Drugs
Club Drugs
Hallucinogens
Methamphetamine
Painkillers
Prescription Drugs

*For a complete list of titles please visit www.referencepointpress.com.

COMPACT *Research*

Diet Drugs

Peggy J. Parks

Drugs

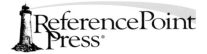
ReferencePoint
Press®

San Diego, CA

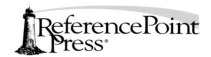

© 2014 ReferencePoint Press, Inc.
Printed in the United States

For more information, contact:
ReferencePoint Press, Inc.
PO Box 27779
San Diego, CA 92198
www.ReferencePointPress.com

Picture credits:
Cover: iStockphoto.com
A. Guillotte: 33–35, 47–49, 61–63, 75, 76
Thinkstock Images: 13, 18

LIBRARY OF CONGRESS CATALOGING-IN-PUBLICATION DATA

Parks, Peggy J., 1951– author.
 Diet drugs : part of the compact research series / by Peggy J. Parks.
  pages cm. -- (Compact research)
 Audience: Grade 9 to 12.
 Includes bibliographical references and index.
 ISBN-13: 978-1-60152-518-5 (hardback)
 ISBN-10: 1-60152-518-4 (hardback)
1. Appetite depressants--Miscellanea. 2. Weight loss preparations--Side effects--Miscellanea.
3. Weight loss preparations industry--Miscellanea. I. Title.
 RM332.3.P37 2014
 615.7'39--dc23
                                                    2013021407

Contents

Foreword

> **"Where is the knowledge we have lost in information?"**

—T.S. Eliot, "The Rock."

As modern civilization continues to evolve, its ability to create, store, distribute, and access information expands exponentially. The explosion of information from all media continues to increase at a phenomenal rate. By 2020 some experts predict the worldwide information base will double every seventy-three days. While access to diverse sources of information and perspectives is paramount to any democratic society, information alone cannot help people gain knowledge and understanding. Information must be organized and presented clearly and succinctly in order to be understood. The challenge in the digital age becomes not the creation of information, but how best to sort, organize, enhance, and present information.

ReferencePoint Press developed the *Compact Research* series with this challenge of the information age in mind. More than any other subject area today, researching current issues can yield vast, diverse, and unqualified information that can be intimidating and overwhelming for even the most advanced and motivated researcher. The *Compact Research* series offers a compact, relevant, intelligent, and conveniently organized collection of information covering a variety of current topics ranging from illegal immigration and deforestation to diseases such as anorexia and meningitis.

The series focuses on three types of information: objective single-author narratives, opinion-based primary source quotations, and facts and statistics. The clearly written objective narratives provide context and reliable background information. Primary source quotes are carefully selected and cited, exposing the reader to differing points of view, and facts and statistics sections aid the reader in evaluating perspectives. Presenting these key types of information creates a richer, more balanced learning experience.

For better understanding and convenience, the series enhances information by organizing it into narrower topics and adding design features that make it easy for a reader to identify desired content. For example, in *Compact Research: Illegal Immigration*, a chapter covering the economic impact of illegal immigration has an objective narrative explaining the various ways the economy is impacted, a balanced section of numerous primary source quotes on the topic, followed by facts and full-color illustrations to encourage evaluation of contrasting perspectives.

The ancient Roman philosopher Lucius Annaeus Seneca wrote, "It is quality rather than quantity that matters." More than just a collection of content, the *Compact Research* series is simply committed to creating, finding, organizing, and presenting the most relevant and appropriate amount of information on a current topic in a user-friendly style that invites, intrigues, and fosters understanding.

Diet Drugs at a Glance

The Obesity Problem

Many weight-loss experts say the need for diet drugs is great because 78 million people in the United States are obese and another one-third are overweight.

Diet Drugs Defined

Diet drugs may be over-the-counter or prescription medications, as well as dietary supplements that are said to promote weight loss.

Types of Diet Drugs

Two main types of diet drugs are appetite suppressants, which trick the body into believing it is not hungry, and fat-absorption inhibitors, which prevent the body from breaking down and absorbing about 25 percent of fat in foods.

Diet-Drug Users

Weight-loss specialists recommend that only people who are obese or seriously overweight use weight-loss drugs, but surveys have shown that the drugs are used by millions of people who do not fit that description.

Oversight of Supplements

Under the 1994 Dietary Supplement Health and Education Act, manufacturers of dietary supplements do not need FDA approval before marketing their products, which means the FDA does not ensure the supplements' potency, purity, safety, or effectiveness.

Effectiveness

Although miracle cures for weight loss do not exist, many people have achieved good results by combining healthy diet, exercise, and a combination of two diet drugs prescribed by a physician.

Side Effects

Depending on the type, diet drugs have been associated with such side effects as anxiety, drowsiness, headaches, excessive thirst, and constipation.

Health Risks

Some of the risks associated with prescription diet drugs include increased heart rate and elevated chance of stroke; some weight-loss supplements have been linked to increased heart rate and high blood pressure.

Diet-Drug Fraud

According to the Federal Trade Commission (FTC), as the demand for diet drugs has grown, fraudulent claims and diet-drug scams have grown proportionately.

Overview

66Whether it's a pill, patch, or cream, there's no shortage of ads promising quick and easy weight loss without diet or exercise. But the claims just aren't true, and some of these products could even hurt your health.99

—Federal Trade Commission, a government agency that exists to protect American consumers from fraud and unfair business practices and to ensure fair competition.

66As with other chronic conditions, such as diabetes or high blood pressure, the use of prescription medications may be appropriate for some people who are overweight or obese.99

—National Institute of Diabetes and Digestive and Kidney Diseases, which conducts and supports medical research to improve people's health and quality of life.

During the summer of 2012 the US Food and Drug Administration (FDA) approved two new diet drugs: Belviq and Qsymia. This was a significant development because it was the first time in thirteen years that the FDA had approved any medication for the treatment of obesity. Also notable was the fact that both drugs had previously been rejected by the agency. Belviq, which was formerly known as Lorqess, was rejected in 2010 after testing showed that it caused breast cancer in lab animals. That same year Qsymia's predecessor (Qnexa) was also rejected by the FDA. It was shown to increase heart rate, and if taken by pregnant women the drug increased the risk of birth defects.

Two years after the drugs were rejected, the FDA changed its position and decided to approve them both. Because this happened without any changes to the drug formulas, a number of medical providers opposed the FDA action, at least until further testing could be done. One physician who was particularly outspoken was Sidney Wolfe, the director of the health research group Public Citizen. "It's either magical or delusional thinking to believe that a drug will turn off hunger without hitting other targets where it will do harm," says Wolfe. "Doctors and patients are desperate for a quick fix. They are desperate to the point where they are willing to risk patients' lives."[1]

The Obesity Epidemic

Supporters of diet drugs acknowledge that there are risks involved for anyone who takes them. They point out, however, that obesity also carries severe health risks, and it has reached epidemic proportions in the United States. "Too many Americans are fat and getting fatter," says Sandra Adamson Fryhofer, a physician from Atlanta, Georgia. "It has to stop."[2] According to the Centers for Disease Control and Prevention (CDC), 78 million American adults are obese and another one-third are overweight. These categories are determined based on people's body mass index (BMI), which is a measure of weight in relation to height. For instance, someone with a BMI of 18.5 to 24.9 is considered to be of normal weight. Those whose body mass index is between 25 and 29.9 are considered overweight, and obesity is a BMI of 30 or higher.

> " Supporters of diet drugs acknowledge that there are risks involved for anyone who takes them. They point out, however, that obesity also carries severe health risks, and it has reached epidemic proportions in the United States. "

Of particular concern to health officials is the disturbing number of children and adolescents who are overweight or obese. In a study published in January 2012 researchers found that 12.1 percent of children aged two to five were obese—more than 5 million girls and 7 million boys. Kelly Brownell, director of Yale University's Rudd Center for Food Policy & Obesity, offers her thoughts: "The numbers in children are particularly alarming because they seem to be growing, and those children tend to track into their adult life with weight problems in those years, as well."[3]

What Are Diet Drugs?

Loosely defined, the term *diet drugs* refers to any medications or supplements that are intended to help people lose weight. They come in a variety of forms, including tablets, capsules, liquids, or powders. Depending on the type, diet drugs may be purchased over the counter at pharmacies or the health and beauty departments of grocery stores, as well as ordered through websites or obtained with a doctor's prescription. When physicians recommend diet drugs to their patients, these are typically drugs that have been approved by the FDA and can be obtained only with a prescription. This is different from the hundreds of varieties of weight-loss supplements, none of which have been subjected to rigorous testing—which means that health officials have no way of knowing if they are safe or effective.

> **Most physicians strongly emphasize that the only people who should take diet drugs are those who are obese or seriously overweight.**

Physicians who prescribe diet drugs to patients who are obese or seriously overweight emphasize that the drugs do not magically make people thin. Rather, the drugs should be viewed as one component of a weight-loss program that includes a healthy diet and increased physical activity. The goal for this approach is twofold: for the person to lose weight, while at the same time developing a healthier lifestyle that will help prevent him or her from gaining the weight back. The Mayo Clinic writes these cautionary words: "The reality is that there's no magic bullet for losing weight. Eat healthy, low-calorie foods, watch portion sizes and be physically active. It's not magic, but it works."[4]

Types of Diet Drugs

Diet drugs perform in different ways, depending on the ingredients they contain and what they have been designed to do. Appetite suppressants, for instance, trick the body into believing it is not hungry by affecting

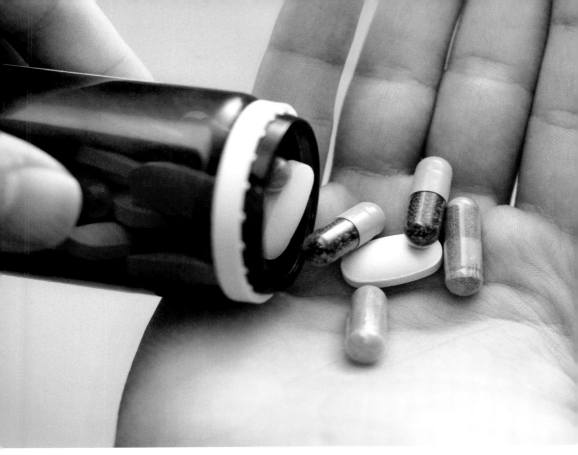

Some diet drugs can be purchased only with a doctor's prescription, while others are sold over the counter as weight-loss supplements. Whether one uses diet drugs or not, exercise and healthy diet are considered essential parts of any weight-loss program.

neurotransmitters, which are chemical messengers that facilitate communication between brain cells. One example is norepinephrine (also called noradrenaline), a neurotransmitter that increases heart rate, triggers the release of glucose from storage in the body, and affects appetite. The diet drug Qsymia is designed to increase levels of norepinephrine in the brain, thereby reducing hunger and increasing satiety, or feelings of being full.

Another type of diet drug is the fat-absorption inhibitor, sometimes called a "fat blocker." These drugs promote weight loss by preventing the body from breaking down and absorbing about 25 percent of fat in foods, which reduces the number of calories a user absorbs. An example of this type of drug is orlistat, which is available by prescription under the name Xenical or in a much weaker, over-the-counter version called Alli. Orlistat works by disabling lipase, an enzyme found in the digestive tract that helps break down dietary fat so it can be used or stored for energy. When fat is not broken down, the body cannot absorb it, meaning that fewer calories are taken in. The undigested fat travels through the intestines and is eliminated during bowel movements.

Who Uses Diet Drugs?

Most physicians strongly emphasize that the only people who should take diet drugs are those who are obese or seriously overweight. The drugs are also acceptable for use by people who are moderately overweight but suffer from conditions such as high blood pressure or diabetes. The National Institute of Diabetes and Digestive and Kidney Diseases (NIDDK) writes: "Prescription weight-loss medications should be used only by patients who are at increased medical risk because of their weight. They should not be used for 'cosmetic' weight loss."[5]

Despite what the NIDDK and other health-related organizations recommend, however, surveys have consistently shown that diet-drug use is not limited to those who are obese. Included in this group, as revealed in the 2012 Youth Risk Behavior survey conducted by CDC researchers, are millions of teenagers. The survey found that 5.1 percent of teens had taken diet pills, powders, or liquids without a doctor's advice to lose weight or keep from gaining weight during the previous month. A breakdown by gender found that from 5.2 to 6.7 percent of the teens who took weight-loss drugs or supplements were girls, and among boys the prevalence ranged from 3.6 to 5 percent.

Early Weight-Loss Drugs

The quest to be thin is a relatively new phenomenon that did not exist until the early 1900s. Throughout prior centuries plumpness was not typically frowned upon; in fact, people who had robust bodies (and equally robust appetites) were viewed as being in good health. The first "fat reducer" drug was named Rengo. Introduced in 1902 by Frank J. Kellogg, the patriarch of the Kellogg cereal dynasty, the product contained thyroid extract as well as a number of other questionable substances and was eventually found to disrupt heart rhythm and weaken the heart muscle. Because this led to users developing high blood pressure, stroke, and cardiac arrest, US health officials removed the drug from the market.

In the 1930s doctors began to prescribe amphetamines for people who needed to lose weight. These drugs are known as stimulants because they stimulate the central nervous system, which causes metabolism to speed up and more calories to be burned. As a result, amphetamines were found to be effective as weight-loss drugs, but there were many problems associated with their use. Side effects included abnormally fast heart rate, altered mood, and chronic insomnia. Also, many people who took the drugs to promote weight loss became seriously addicted to them. Once these negative effects became known, doctors were not so quick to prescribe amphetamines for their patients.

One drug that appeared to be promising for weight loss was discovered during the 1930s by three physicians from Stanford University. Maurice L. Tainter ,Windsor C. Cutting, and A.B. Stockton observed that an industrial chemical known as dinitrophenol (DNP) could speed up metabolism. They theorized that when people took DNP, food energy was dissipated as heat rather than converted into fat. If this was true, the chemical could potentially be a successful weight-loss drug.

> " In the United States, drugs can be sold only if they have been approved by the FDA, although what constitutes a 'drug' depends on its intended use. "

By 1934, however, the three physicians had become concerned about DNP, as medical journalist Kathleen Donnelly writes: "In the year since the publication of their first paper, they estimated at least 100,000 people in the United States had taken DNP. The worry? DNP was showing up in easily available weight-loss medicines. Drs. Tainter and Cutting fretted that people were taking too much. They already knew of at least two deaths due to fatally high fevers possibly brought on by overdoses of DNP."[6] Health officials conducted an investigation and found a link between DNP and permanent blindness, as well as deaths due to high fever. In 1938, when the Federal Food, Drug, and Cosmetic Act gave the FDA the power to remove drugs from the marketplace, DNP was among the first to go.

How Diet Drugs Are Regulated

In the United States, drugs can be sold only if they have been approved by the FDA, although what constitutes a "drug" depends on its intended use. Substances that are created for the purpose of curing, treating, or preventing disease, or to lessen the symptoms of disease, fall under the category of drugs, as the regulatory consulting firm FDA Imports explains: "Almost any ingested or topical or injectable product that, through its label or labeling (including internet websites, promotional pamphlets, and other marketing material), is claimed to be beneficial for such uses will be regulated by FDA as a drug."[7]

Pharmaceutical companies who want to market new drugs must obtain the FDA's approval before doing so. This includes prescription drugs as well as those that are available over the counter, which the FDA refers to as nonprescription drugs. Drug safety specialist Susan Thaul writes: "To get that approval, the manufacturer must demonstrate the drug's safety and effectiveness according to criteria specified in law and agency regulations, ensure that its manufacturing plant passes FDA inspection, and obtain FDA approval for the drug's labeling—a term that includes all written material about the drug, including, for example, packaging, prescribing information for physicians, and patient brochures."[8]

> " Diet-drug advertising is notorious for its lofty claims—promises of amazing results that are exactly what overweight and obese people desperately want to believe. "

The regulatory procedure for dietary supplements, including those that purportedly help people lose weight, is not the same as for drugs. These supplements may be vitamins, minerals, herbs, amino acids, or other substances that are designed to complete a diet or to make up for a dietary deficiency. There is no requirement for premarket testing for supplement safety and effectiveness, and supplement manufacturers are not required to register their products with the FDA or report adverse events from product usage. As a result, the FDA does not ensure the potency, purity, safety, or effectiveness, of dietary supplements. This is important for consumers to know because they may assume that all weight-loss products sold in American stores are safe and effective—and that is not necessarily the case. If the FDA has suspicions about safety, the agency launches an investigation and, if warranted, takes steps to have the product removed from circulation. "However," says the FDA, "it is much easier for a firm to get a product on the market than it is for FDA to take a product off the market."[9]

How Effective Are Diet Drugs?

Diet-drug advertising is notorious for its lofty claims—promises of amazing results that are exactly what overweight and obese people desperately want to believe. Public health officials, however, warn that quick-fix solutions for weight loss do not exist. Canadian obesity specialists Yoni Freedhoff and Arya M. Sharma write: "The $50 billion North American weight-loss industry comprises a morass of fantastical claims of products and programs promising quick, easy, long-lasting results. Given this wealth of magical weight-loss aids, why is obesity still a problem? Perhaps because magic exists solely within consumers' hopes and dreams, which many commercial weight-loss providers happily exploit."[10]

Because overweight people are so eager for easy, painless ways of losing weight, they are especially vulnerable to enticing marketing messages. For that reason, obesity specialists often become irritated when famous celebrities endorse weight-loss products. This happened in September 2011, when reality TV star Nicole Polizzi (better known as Snooki) publicly announced that she had lost seventeen pounds. Polizzi said that her weight loss was due to a combination of dieting, exercise, and taking the herbal dietary supplement Zantrex-3. She went on to announce that she would become the national spokesperson for the Zantrex-3 "extreme

> **All drugs and supplements, whether they are purchased over the counter at pharmacies and grocery stores, ordered from websites, or obtained through a doctor's prescription, carry the risk of side effects.**

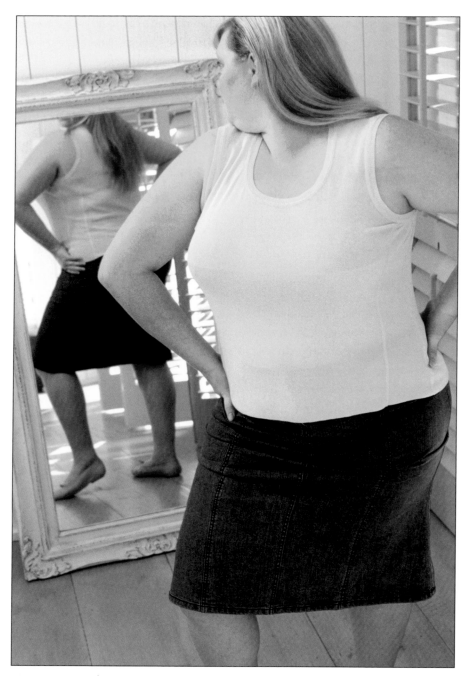

Millions of Americans are obese or overweight and searching for ways to lose weight. Experts say those who turn to unproven dietary supplements may be wasting money and risking their health.

energy" fat-burning pill. Upon hearing the news, Keith Ayoob of the Albert Einstein College of Medicine wasted no time in expressing his disapproval. "This is outrageous," Ayoob says. "It's a perfect example of bad endorsement. It's a quick fix, potentially a dangerous one, and celebs may have a high profile, but they're often not very credible sources."[11]

Diet-Drug Side Effects

All drugs and supplements, whether they are purchased over the counter at pharmacies and grocery stores, ordered from websites, or obtained through a doctor's prescription, carry the risk of side effects. Diet drugs are no exception, which is why there are not many FDA-approved choices for patients. Neurobiologist and obesity researcher Stephan Guyenet writes: "There are very few obesity drugs currently approved for use in the US—not because effective drugs don't exist, but because the FDA has judged that the side effects of existing drugs are unacceptable."[12] Depending on the type, diet drugs have been associated with insomnia, nervousness/anxiety, dizziness, drowsiness, headaches, excessive thirst, dry mouth, and constipation, among other side effects.

Since they were first introduced, the fat blockers Xenical and Alli have been marketed as weight-loss drugs that must be used in conjunction with a low-fat diet—specifically, a diet that contains less than forty-two grams of fat per day. Package inserts clearly state that if users ignore this advice, they risk unpredictable—and embarrassing—loose, runny stools and oily spotting. David Sarwer, director of clinical services at the University of Pennsylvania School of Medicine's Center for Weight Loss and Eating Disorders, says that learning the hard way to heed manufacturers' warnings is not necessarily a bad lesson. He explains: "It forces you to eat a lower-fat diet—if you don't, you're violently penalized for not doing so. When [users] eat a little too much fat, they'll learn not to do it again."[13]

What Are the Health Risks of Diet Drugs?

Along with side effects, which can be unpleasant and uncomfortable, diet drugs have been associated with serious health problems. People who take Belviq, for instance, are warned of the possibility of hallucinations, uncontrolled muscle spasms, suicidal thoughts, and changes in heart rate and blood pressure. One of Qsymia's active ingredients is phentermine, a stimulant drug that many physicians believe can be dangerous. A June

2013 article in the *UC Berkeley Wellness Letter* explains: "Notably, it can cause spikes in heart rate. It also increases the risk of kidney stones, glaucoma, metabolic acidosis [a buildup of acid in the body], and low blood sugar."[14] The article goes on to say that Qysmia's other active chemical, topiramate, can negatively affect mood and has been linked to memory and concentration problems.

> "As the obesity epidemic has continued to grow in severity, the demand for diet drugs has soared—and so have fraudulent claims and diet-drug scams."

Even though prescription diet drugs like Belviq and Qysmia can be risky, they are regulated by the FDA, so their use is controlled and monitored. The same is not true, however, for the multitude of dietary supplements available for sale on the Internet. One example is Slimming Beauty Bitter Orange Slimming Capsules, a weight-loss supplement sold through a number of websites. The advertising and product labels claim that the supplement is 100 percent herbal, a natural product that is safe for use even by young children. But the label neglects to state that the pills contain sibutramine, a powerful stimulant that can legally be sold only with a doctor's prescription. In October 2010, when the FDA learned about the availability of the Slimming Beauty capsules, it issued a warning that strongly dissuaded consumers from buying the product.

How Big a Problem Is Diet-Drug Fraud?

As the obesity epidemic has continued to grow in severity, the demand for diet drugs has soared—and so have fraudulent claims and diet-drug scams. According to the FDA, a health product is fraudulent if it is deceptively promoted as being effective against a certain condition (such as obesity) but has not been scientifically proved to be safe and effective for that purpose.

In February 2011 the FDA issued several warnings about fake weight-loss products that were being marketed as legitimate FDA-approved substances. Undercover FDA agents working in Denver, Colorado, arrested a thirty-one-year-old Chinese man named Shengyang Zhou, who was selling counterfeit Alli. He was trafficking and importing the drug into the United States from China, as well as marketing it on his website and through the online auction site eBay. A number of people got sick after taking the counterfeit drugs, including an emergency room doctor from Houston, Texas, who suffered a mild stroke.

A Difficult Battle

Diet drugs are a controversial issue. Medical professionals who are opposed to them say that obese and overweight people need to lose weight the *correct* way: by modifying their diets and becoming more physically active rather than relying on drugs to do the work for them. Opponents also contend that taking drugs is risky and people should be discouraged from doing so. Supporters do not disagree about the importance of a healthier lifestyle, nor do they deny that there are risks involved. They are convinced, however, that the benefits of diet drugs far outweigh the risks, and they emphasize that weight-loss medicines are not intended to replace healthy eating and exercise. Rather, they should be viewed as one more tool to help people lose weight and live happier, healthier lives.

What Are Diet Drugs?

❝It's too bad there is no similar societal and public health commitment in our society to marketing healthy food and lifestyle choices as there is to developing drugs for weight loss.❞

—Judy Stone, a physician and clinical researcher from Cumberland, Maryland.

❝Most people cannot achieve long term weight loss by diet and exercise alone.❞

—Steven R. Smith, professor and scientific director of the Florida Hospital/Sanford-Burnham Translational Research Institute for Metabolism and Diabetes.

After numerous unsuccessful attempts to lose the extra weight she had gained while being out of work, Jennifer Sibley was definitely ready for a new approach. In terms of prescription diet drugs, she found few options from which to choose, so she decided to try a practice known as "combo-pilling." As the name implies, combo-pilling involves taking a combination of two different drugs. The thinking behind this practice is that the drugs will work together and be more effective at achieving weight loss as a pair than either would alone. The two drugs Sibley chose were the appetite suppressant phentermine, which she ordered from a website, and topiramate (brand name Topamax), a drug for treating epilepsy and migraine headaches that she had gotten with a prescription. She did not seek medical advice or supervision for her combo-pilling–weight-loss attempt—and she soon realized what a mistake that was.

Sibley, a former advertising executive who had been unemployed for a year, was in the middle of an intensive job search when she began taking the drugs. After starting her diet-drug regimen she began to suffer from peculiar, disturbing side effects. During a phone interview she could not focus on what the prospective employer was saying, and at times her mind went completely blank. After losing out on that job, and then a second one that required a face-to-face interview, Sibley knew that the drugs were affecting her brain. "That's when I stopped taking the pills," she says. "I came home and thought, it's not worth it. These drugs are making me nutty."[15]

Drug Combos

Sibley made the unwise decision to create her own drug combination, but the practice of combo-pilling is not uncommon among physicians who treat overweight and obese patients. Although the phentermine/topiramate combination is now contained in Qsymia, long before that drug was on the market doctors had been prescribing the two drugs together. They were also writing prescriptions for other drug combinations in an effort to help patients lose weight. In a July 2012 *Wall Street Journal* article, health journalist Melinda Beck writes: "Some obesity specialists, including those at prestigious medical centers, have been prescribing medications to help patients lose weight for decades, both on and off-label."[16]

The term "off-label" refers to the practice of prescribing drugs differently from what the FDA has officially approved. For example, a drug may be prescribed for a different disease or medical condition than originally intended, given in a different dose, or prescribed for longer periods of time. Off-label drug use is an acceptable and common practice among health care professionals. Says Beck: "Physicians can legally prescribe medications for uses not specifically approved

> " As the name implies, combo-pilling involves taking a combination of two different drugs. "

by the FDA. But most obesity doctors do so cautiously given the history of diet pills removed from the market due to serious side effects including death."[17] In addition to topiramate, some other non-diet drugs that physicians prescribe off-label for weight loss include the anticonvulsant drug zonisamide; a diabetes medication called metformin;

and bupropion, an antidepressant that is marketed under the names of Wellbutrin and Zyban.

Michael Anchors, an obesity specialist whose practice is in Gaithersburg, Maryland, created an effective weight-loss-drug combo for which he holds a patent. Known as phen-Pro, Anchors's drug cocktail contains phentermine and the antidepressant Prozac. He regularly prescribes it for his patients who want to lose weight—and not only those who are obese. When asked how overweight a patient must be in order for him to treat him or her with his phen-Pro diet-drug cocktail, Anchors answers: "A pound," and then goes on to say, "Seriously. If you're even one pound more than you want to be and you haven't been successful in losing it, why shouldn't I help? I mean, these are safe medicines now. I can't think of a reason not to."[18]

> In addition to topiramate, some other non-diet drugs that physicians prescribe off-label for weight loss include the anticonvulsant drug zonisamide; a diabetes medication called metformin; and bupropion, an antidepressant that is marketed under the names of Wellbutrin and Zyban.

Yet Anchors goes much further than merely prescribing drugs for his weight-loss patients. He stresses to them the importance of lifestyle changes, including adopting healthier eating habits. "A pill can make a person less hungry," he says, "but it can't tell them how to eat."[19] In his practice Anchors uses a weight-loss regimen that includes drug therapy combined with nutrition education and exercise. Like other weight-loss specialists, he is convinced that this sort of comprehensive approach is the only way to maintain the weight loss in the long run.

One of Anchors's patients is Marianne Greenhouse, who weighed more than three hundred pounds when she first consulted with Anchors. Within six months of changing her diet, becoming more active, and taking the phen-Pro combo, she had lost fifty pounds. "Now I feel like I have a future,"[20] says Greenhouse.

The Fen-Phen Fiasco

Although prescribing combinations of drugs for weight loss is widespread today, it has a rocky history. The first health care professional known to experiment with the practice was Michael Weintraub, who during the 1980s was a pharmacologist at the University of Rochester in Rochester, New York. Weintraub read about two appetite suppressants: fenfluramine, which caused feelings of satiety, and the stimulant drug phentermine. Alone, neither of these drugs was believed to be very effective at helping with weight loss, largely because of side effects: One caused drowsiness and the other caused jitteriness. "What struck me," says Weintraub, "was that the side effects were this and that with one of the drugs, and the opposite—that and this—with the other." Weintraub became curious about what would happen if the two drugs were combined—if the side effects of one might cancel out the side effects of the other. "I decided to try them together,"[21] he says.

In 1992 Weintraub and his colleagues published the results of a long-term study that was funded by the National Heart, Lung, and Blood Institute. The study involved 121 adults who were between 30 percent and 80 percent over their ideal weight. Participants were randomly divided into two groups: a medication group whose members were given a cocktail of fenfluramine and phentermine (known as fen-phen) and a group whose members were given a placebo, meaning dummy pills containing no active medication. At the beginning of the study all participants began a program of exercise, dieting, and behavior modification (learning to change one's thoughts, fears, and feelings), and this continued throughout the entire study period.

> As the obesity problem in the United States has continued to worsen, scientists have aggressively pursued research to find effective, safe weight-loss drugs.

The research team's findings were quite profound. Participants who took the fen-phen drug combination lost about 16 percent of their initial weight, compared with the placebo group whose average weight loss was less than 5 percent. In her book *Dispensing with the Truth*, author Alicia Mundy writes: "What followed was a media frenzy touting fen-phen as an obesity wonder drug, including a 1995 profile in the women's magazine *Allure*. By 1997, between 6 and 7 million American women had taken fen-phen, along with its prescriptive sister Redux. And it was not just the obese who were gobbling these diet drugs—those who wanted to quickly shed 10 to 15 pounds begged their doctors for a prescription."[22]

With her reference to "Redux," Mundy is talking about a hybrid drug called dexfenfluramine, which combined fenfluramine and phentermine in one pill and was approved by the FDA in 1996. In that one year, physicians wrote 18 million fen-phen prescriptions each month—but the fen-phen craze was short-lived. In August 1997 Mayo Clinic physician Heidi Connelly published an article in the *New England Journal of Medicine* about heart valve abnormalities among twenty-four women who were taking the combination of fenfluramine and phentermine. Connelly noted that doctors had not observed this problem before meaning that it was likely a direct result of the drugs. Following the publication of her article, the FDA learned of another seventy-five cases of heart valve disease among patients who took fen-phen drugs and/or Redux.

On September 15, 1997, the FDA removed both Redux and fenfluramine from the market. In a public statement, the agency's lead deputy commissioner Michael A. Friedman said: "These findings call for prompt action. The data we have obtained indicate that fenfluramine, and the chemically closely related dexfenfluramine, present an unacceptable risk at this time to patients who take them."[23] Phentermine remained available because it had not been associated with heart problems and was deemed to be a safe drug.

Phen Popularity

Today, phentermine is still regularly prescribed by doctors for weight loss. In fact, the NIDDK says that it is the most commonly prescribed appetite suppressant in the United States. Phentermine is available as tablets or extended-release capsules and is usually taken as a single daily dose in the morning, although some physicians may prescribe it to be taken up to three times a day. According to the National Institutes of Health, most people take phentermine for three to six weeks and are then evaluated by their physician to see how well the drug is working.

Some people order the drug online, which medical professionals strongly discourage because it is extremely risky.

Piper Miguelgorry, an environmental researcher from Folsom, California, had gained a lot of weight after three pregnancies and was having a hard time losing the extra pounds. She visited a weight-loss center where phentermine was part of her individualized plan, along with a high-protein, low-carbohydrate diet. "Much to my surprise," she says, "I lost 50 pounds."[24] Miguelgorry credits phentermine with helping to reduce her cravings for carbohydrates and is so happy with her weight loss that she plans to continue taking the drug indefinitely. In addition to being thinner, she has seen other improvements in her health as well, such as lowering her cholesterol by half and overcoming type-2 diabetes.

A Promising Finding

As the obesity problem in the United States has continued to worsen, scientists have aggressively pursued research to find effective, safe weight-loss drugs. According to a study published in the August 8, 2012, issue of the medical science journal *Cell Metabolism*, a new drug known as JD5037 might be just what they are looking for.

Researchers from the National Institute on Alcohol Abuse and Alcoholism (NIAAA) created JD5037 to increase the body's sensitivity to leptin, an appetite-suppressing hormone. It is well known among scientists that obese people become desensitized to leptin due to activity among cannabinoid receptors, or molecules in the brain that help facilitate various brain and body functions. Prior studies had shown that blocking the receptors could lead to weight loss, and a drug called rimonabant was developed to block these receptors. The drug was marketed in the United Kingdom but taken out of circulation in 2008 after it was found to cause serious psychiatric side effects including anxiety, depression, and suicidal thoughts.

> " For people who want to lose weight, diet drugs can be one more tool to help them achieve their goal. "

For the NIAAA study, laboratory mice were intentionally made obese by being fed a high-fat diet. One group was treated with JD5037 daily for about a month, and the mice in the group lost 28 percent of their body weight, reaching the weight of normal-sized mice. In addition, they showed little interest in the high-fat diet that had made them obese, and showed no obvious side effects from the drug. "This is a very promising finding," says NIAAA director Kenneth R. Warren. "Obesity is one of our most pressing public health problems, for which new therapies are urgently needed."[25] The NIAAA researchers cannot say for sure if they will see the same result when people, rather than mice, are treated with JD5037. They are hopeful that they will and continue to pursue further studies with humans.

Challenges and Hope

For people who want to lose weight, diet drugs can be one more tool to help them achieve their goal. There are few FDA-approved prescription diet drugs, but physicians often prescribe combinations of off-label medications, and many of these have proved to be effective. Yet despite these options, there is no miraculous solution, no magical concoction that is guaranteed to melt fat and ensure svelte bodies without effort. As scientists continue to pursue research, promising new drugs are becoming more likely.

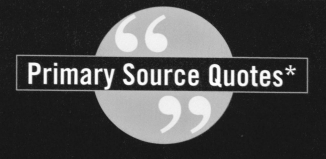

Primary Source Quotes*

What Are Diet Drugs?

66 The American obsession with physical image and an ideal size two model has driven a number of individuals to engage in unhealthy activities, including the excessive use of diet pills. 99

—Elements Behavioral Health, "Diet Pill Addiction: It Isn't Worth the Weight," July 5, 2011. www.treatmentcenters.net.

Headquartered in Long Beach, California, Elements Behavioral Health offers specialized addiction treatment programs at a number of locations.

66 There are some crazy, wacky diets that take losing weight to an extreme. Presently the most popular diet of all is the prescription-drug diet. 99

—Vincent Bellonzi, *Health Recklessly Abandoned.* Garden City, NY: Morgan James, 2013, p. 12.

Bellonzi is a doctor of chiropractic medicine and a certified clinical nutritionist at the Austin Wellness Clinic in Austin, Texas.

* Editor's Note: While the definition of a primary source can be narrowly or broadly defined, for the purposes of Compact Research, a primary source consists of: 1) results of original research presented by an organization or researcher; 2) eyewitness accounts of events, personal experience, or work experience; 3) first-person editorials offering pundits' opinions; 4) government officials presenting political plans and/or policies; 5) representatives of organizations presenting testimony or policy.

Primary Source Quotes

“There is no shortcut to weight loss. Eating wholesome food in moderate amounts, drinking water, and exercising are the answer to sensible weight loss and optimal health—not drugs.”

—Wendy Ford, interview with author, May 16, 2013.

Ford is a doctor of chiropractic medicine from Hatboro, Pennsylvania.

“So-called weight-loss drugs are huge business, but they’re going from bad to worse.”

—Alliance for Natural Health, “Diet Pills That ‘Help’ Depression—with Confusion, Hostility, and Heart Problems,” March 8, 2011. www.anh-usa.org.

The Alliance for Natural Health is an advocacy organization that advocates a healthy diet and lifestyle and favors alternative medicine over drugs, surgery, and other conventional techniques.

“One thing that the world has way too many of is diet pills. They are everywhere, on TV infomercials, all over TV commercials, in magazines, and they can be found at any local drug store or nutrition center quite easily.”

—Seacliff Recovery Center, “Diet Pill Abuse,” December 29, 2012. http://seacliffrecovery.com.

Seacliff Recovery Center is a full-service rehabilitation facility located in Huntington Beach, California.

“Most weight-loss pills contain multiple ingredients, such as herbs, botanicals, vitamins, minerals, and even caffeine or laxatives.”

—Mayo Clinic, “Over-the-Counter Weight-Loss Pills: Do They Work?,” February 11, 2012. www.mayoclinic.com.

Mayo Clinic is a world-renowned health care facility headquartered in Rochester, Minnesota.

“The FDA continues to warn consumers, but diet pills aren't illegal and new varieties sprout like dandelions.”

—Cynthia Sass, “The Dangers of Diet Pills,” blog, *Shape*, November 4, 2011. www.shape.com.

Sass is a registered dietician who holds master's degrees in both nutrition science and public health.

“Phentermine may be recommended as part of an overall weight-loss plan if you're significantly over-weight—not if you want to lose just a few pounds.”

—Donald Hensrud, “Is Phentermine a Good Option for Weight Loss?,” Mayo Clinic, October 22, 2011. www.mayoclinic.com.

Hensrud is a preventive medicine and nutrition specialist at Mayo Clinic in Rochester, Minnesota.

What Are Diet Drugs?

- A study published in June 2011 by researchers from the University of Minnesota found that **20 percent** of young adult women used binge eating, fasting, diet pills, or other extreme measures to control their weight.

- According to Pieter A. Cohen, an internist with Cambridge Health Alliance and an assistant professor of medicine at Harvard Medical School, **15 percent** of American adults use weight-loss supplements.

- As of June 2013 the only over-the-counter weight-loss drug that had been approved by the FDA was the **fat-blocker drug Alli.**

- A Youth Risk Behavior Surveillance survey that was published in June 2012 found that **5.1 percent** of students in the United States had taken diet pills, powders, or liquids—without a doctor's advice—to lose weight or keep from gaining weight.

- According to health care experts from the University of California at Berkeley, as of June 2013 more than **two hundred diet drugs** were in development.

- According to Yale University clinical neurologist Steven Novella, a 2010 analysis of eighty-one weight-loss supplements marketed in Hong Kong found that **sixty-one** of them contained two or more **pharmaceutical agents**, and two supplements contained six different drugs.

High School Students Who Took Weight-Loss Products in the Past 30 Days

In a study that was published in June 2012, students in ninth through twelfth grades from schools throughout the United States were asked questions about their health-risk behaviors. As this graph shows, teenage girls in all grades used diet pills, powders, or liquids at higher rates than boys of the same age.

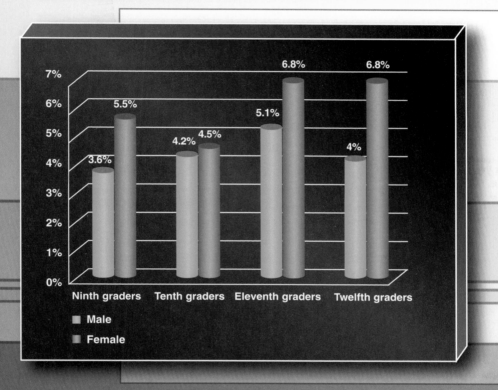

Source: Danice K. Eaton, et al, "Youth Risk Behavioral Surveillance—United States, 2011," *Morbidity and Mortality Weekly Report*, June 8, 2012. www.cdc.gov.

- A study published in June 2011 by researchers from the University of Minnesota found that the use of diet pills more than **tripled** among most groups that were followed over the ten-year period.

Types of Prescription Diet Drugs

Diet drugs are catagorized based on their functions, or how they are designed to work. This diagram shows the types of prescription diet drugs that are currently approved by the Food and Drug Administration (FDA).

Drug (and trade name)	How it works
Diethylpropion (Tenuate)	Decreases appetite, increases feeling of fullness
Lorcaserin (Belviq)	Decreases appetite, increases feeling of fullness
Phentermine (Adipex)	Decreases appetite, increases feeling of fullness
Orlistat (prescription drug: Xenical; over-the-counter: Alli)	Blocks absorption of fat
Phentermine and extended-release topiramate (Qsymia)	Decreases appetite, increases feeling of fullness

Source: Mayo Clinic, "Prescription Weight-Loss Drugs: Can They Help You?," July 27, 2012. www.mayoclinic.com.

- A study published in April 2013 by the market research firm Marketdata found that total sales of all diet- and weight-loss-related products totaled **$61.56 billion** in 2012, with prescription diet drugs representing only one-half percent of the total amount.

- According to the National Institute of Diabetes and Digestive and Kidney Disorders, prescription weight-loss medications should be used only by people whose **body mass index** (BMI) is 30 and above, or whose BMI is at least 27 with an obesity-related condition such as high blood pressure, diabetes, or dyslipidemia (abnormal amounts of fat in the blood).

- The FDA states that the only weight-loss medication approved for longer-term use is **orlistat** (brand names, Xenical and Alli), although its safety and effectiveness have not been established for use beyond two years.

Diet Drugs Are Small Part of Weight-Loss Market

In April 2013 the market research firm Marketdata published a study on the weight-loss and diet market in the United States. Total sales of all diet and weight-loss–related products totaled about $62 billion in 2012, with prescription and over-the-counter diet drugs representing only a fraction of the total amount.

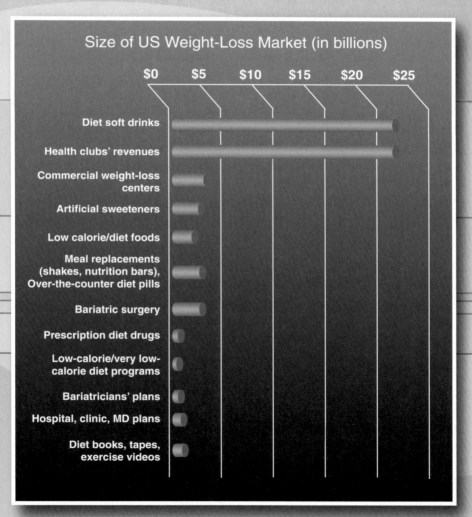

Source: PRWeb, "Weight Loss Market in U.S. Up 1.7% to $61 Billion," April 16, 2013. www.prweb.com.

How Effective Are Diet Drugs?

66Diet drugs don't work, they interfere with the body's metabolism, and don't address the obesity problem in any meaningful way. The only way to lose weight is decrease caloric intake and move more.99

—Wendy Ford, a doctor of chiropractic medicine from Hatboro, Pennsylvania.

66There are useful dietary supplements manufactured with integrity that I do recommend to my private practice clients, but diet pills aren't among them. If something sounds too good to be true it probably is.99

—Cynthia Sass, a registered dietician who holds master's degrees in both nutrition science and public health.

By the time Anne Grauso sought help from weight-loss specialist Louis Aronne, she had grown to hate how she looked. A former svelte model and athlete, Grauso had gotten heavier after having a child and put on more weight while taking fertility treatments in an effort to conceive again. Still, she was not too concerned because she desperately wanted to get pregnant, and that was her focus. She remained unfazed by her weight gain even as she had to keep buying larger and larger sizes because her clothes were too tight. "Of course, I didn't realize I was getting super heavy and I looked like crap,"[26] she says.

The turning point for Grauso came in 2008. Being part of New York City's high society she frequently attended glitzy social events, and her picture often appeared in the *Sunday Styles* section of the *New York Times*. One of those pictures forced her into realizing that she needed to get aggressive about losing weight. "I remember opening the [paper] and seeing a picture of myself at a party and just crying," says Grauso. "It was awful. I thought, 'I need a plan. This isn't me.'"[27]

Same Person, Different Body

Grauso visited Aronne at the Comprehensive Weight Control Program at New York–Presbyterian Hospital, and he developed a personalized weight-loss regimen for her. She began eating a healthier, low-fat diet and drinking plenty of water, while increasing her physical activity to include kickboxing and several other types of exercise. Aronne also gave her a prescription for the drugs Wellbutrin and Topamax (topiramate), which he believed could help her reach her goals. "Medicine helps people do better on a program of diet and exercise," says Aronne. "It's not instead of . . . it's in addition to."[28]

> **Many people have had good luck losing weight with a multipronged approach: changing their diets, becoming more active, and taking drugs that are often prescribed in pairs.**

By the end of a year, after Grauso had faithfully stuck with her weight-loss program, she had lost sixty pounds and dropped five dress sizes. The change was striking—so striking, in fact, that she was often asked if she had had weight-loss surgery. Each time, she shook her head and replied, "I sweat it off." Upon reaching her goal, Grauso felt a sense of pride at how much her hard work had paid off. "I feel like I'm capable of anything," she says. "I can change anything in my life. I've proven that I can. Anything is possible."[29]

Dynamic Duo

Like Grauso, many people have had good luck losing weight with a multipronged approach: changing their diets, becoming more active, and taking drugs that are often prescribed in pairs. Evaluating the effectiveness of the phentermine and topiramate combination was the focus of a study published in April 2011 by researchers from Duke University Medical Center. The study involved 2,487 adults from ninety-three weight-loss centers throughout the United States. All participants were either over-weight or obese and suffered from at least two physical conditions, such as high blood pressure and diabetes. Each was given information about the importance of healthy diet and lifestyle practices.

> "A major reason for the popularity of drug combos is that for years physicians had few choices of diet drugs to prescribe for their overweight and obese patients. "

Participants were randomly assigned to receive one of three treatments once per day: phentermine plus topiramate, a higher dose of the same combination, or a placebo. At the end of the fifty-six-week study period, participants in the lower-dose group lost an average of 18 pounds (8.1 kg) and those in the higher-dose group lost an average of 22 pounds (10 kg). This can be compared with the placebo group, whose members lost an average of 3 pounds (1.4 kg).

According to lead researcher Kishore M. Gadde, who directs the obesity clinical trials program at Duke University Medical Center, the combination of phentermine plus topiramate may be effective because both drugs have several ways of acting on the body to induce weight loss. "When you have a drug with multiple mechanisms of action," he says, "there's a greater chance that it's going to have much more efficacy. The brain has the capacity to find a way to make you eat again if we are just manipulating one small pathway. If you're attacking the appetite centers from a number of different angles, you have potentially greater success."[30]

Clinical Trials

A major reason for the popularity of drug combos is that for years physicians had few choices of diet drugs to prescribe for their overweight and obese patients. Thus, they created custom drug cocktails that were believed to work better than any single drug. So in 2012, when the FDA reversed its earlier position and approved Belviq and Qsymia, it was good news for physicians and patients. The FDA's approval came on the heels of clinical trials that had shown both drugs to be very effective at helping people lose weight.

Belviq (lorcaserin) was tested in three clinical trials conducted at weight-loss centers throughout the United States. The first involved 3,182 adults; the second involved 4,008 adults, and the third involved 604 adults, for a total of 7,794 participants. Everyone in the study was either overweight or obese, and participants in the third group suffered from type 2 diabetes. Members of all groups received individualized counseling for reduced-calorie dieting and exercise at the time of their first dose (Belviq or placebo) as well as every four weeks after that.

At the conclusion of the trials, the researchers found that the average weight loss among participants taking Belviq ranged from 3 to 3.7 percent higher than those who were given a placebo. Among participants without type 2 diabetes, nearly half lost at least 5 percent of their weight compared with 23 percent of patients in the placebo group. In a published report of one of the trials, the researchers write: "Lorcaserin administration for 1 yr in conjunction with diet and exercise counseling to obese and overweight adults was associated with clinically and statistically significant weight loss. Significant decreases in body fat content, waist circumference, and quality of life accompanied the reduction in body weight."[31]

> **Most physicians and obesity experts say they do not recommend weight-loss supplements because evidence that the supplements are effective is sorely lacking.**

The results of clinical trials with Qsymia were even more impressive. The drug (phentermine plus topiramate) was tested in two clinical trials that involved nearly 3,700 obese and overweight patients. Participants were assigned to one of three groups: those who received a low dose of the drug, a higher dose of the drug, or a placebo. At the end of the studies, the average weight loss of patients taking Qsymia ranged from 6.7 percent (low dose) to 8.9 percent (high dose) over those taking a placebo. Specifically, 62 percent of patients taking the lowest dose of the drug and 70 percent on the higher dose lost at least 5 percent of their weight, compared with the 20 percent of participants who were given a placebo.

Beneficial or Bogus?

Of all the weight-loss methods that exist, dietary supplements are among the most controversial. Most physicians and obesity experts say they do not recommend weight-loss supplements because evidence that the supplements are effective is sorely lacking. Says Steven Novella, a clinical neurologist at the Yale University School of Medicine: "Weight loss supplements are a 2.4 billion dollar industry in the US—an industry based entirely on products that do not work, and some of which are not entirely safe. In addition to this financial waste, weight loss supplements distract people from weight loss methods that at least have a chance to be effective (lifestyle changes, regular exercise, calorie control)."[32]

This "effective" method of losing weight is the premise of the reality TV show *The Biggest Loser*. For all the years it has been on the air, the show has emphasized that the only sensible, permanent way to lose weight is through diet and exercise. Because of that, it was disturbing to obesity specialists to learn that two of the show's trainers were touting the benefits of weight-loss supplements. In a March 2013 report on its ThinkProgress blog, the Center for American Progress Action Fund revealed that trainers Bob Harper and Jillian Michaels were promoting their own collection of weight-loss supplements. Michaels touts hers by emphasizing that she would never put her name on something unless she truly believed in its effectiveness. Harper claims that his supplements are unlike anything else that is available.

> " The effectiveness (or lack thereof) of diet drugs is an issue with many variables and no simple answers. "

When it became public that Harper and Michaels were publicly endorsing weight-loss supplements, many experts were furious. The two were accused of using their fame to sell products that were not proved effective and could potentially be harmful. Michaels was sued by four different people who had tried her supplements, although the lawsuits were dismissed. Referring to one of her products that she claims will cleanse the body and rid it of toxins, Indiana University pharmacology professor Lynn Willis states: "This product is an absurdity. It's completely bogus that this would detoxify the gut. Someone takes a laxative and they lose two pounds of water weight, but it will come right back."[33]

An Eye-Opening Study

In March 2012 Oregon State University diet and nutrition professor Melinda Manore announced the findings of a study that focused on dietary supplements. Manore, who is considered an expert in health, nutrition, and weight management has been conducting research for more than twenty-five years. Her study involved an extensive review of literature related to hundreds of weight-loss supplements, and she published it in the *International Journal of Sports Nutrition and Exercise Metabolism*. Manore's conclusion was that weight-loss supplements were ineffective and a waste of money. "Most weight-loss supplements are not worth the money spent on them, and some can be harmful," she says. "If weight loss does occur, the amount is typically around 2 to 3 kilograms (4 to 7 pounds), which is not the type of weight loss most people want."[34]

Manore adds that the biggest problem is unrealistic expectations by the people who want to lose weight and think supplements are the answer. "Consumers don't realize that most weight-loss supplements are tested in the context of a hypocaloric diet, which means people need to reduce the number of calories they are consuming," she says. "They don't want to do that. They just want to take a pill and have the weight melt off without changing diet, physical activity, lifestyle, and environment."[35]

The Green Coffee Bean Diet

On April 9, 2013, researchers giving a presentation at a meeting of the American Chemical Society discussed a family of substances called chlorogenic acids, which occur naturally in apples, cherries, plums, and other fruits, as well as vegetables. The lead presenter was Joe Vinson, a chemistry professor at the University of Scranton in Scranton, Pennsylvania. Vinson explained to the audience that large amounts of these acids have also been discovered in green (meaning unroasted) coffee beans—and when people took an extract of the beans, it helped them lose weight.

Vinson was the lead researcher for a study that involved sixteen participants who were either obese or overweight. They were divided into three groups: a high-dose (1,050 milligrams) green coffee bean extract group, a low-dose (700 milligrams) green coffee bean extract group, and a group whose members were given a placebo. This was what is known as a crossover study, meaning that participants rotated from one group to another, rather than being in the same group for the entire five-month study period. Everyone involved was closely monitored as they ate a healthy low-fat diet and exercised on a regular basis.

At the conclusion of the study, the participants had lost an average of 17 pounds, which represented (on average) a 10.5 percent decrease in overall body weight and a 16 percent decrease in body fat. Although further study may be needed, Vinson believes the weight loss would have been even more significant had all participants received only the higher dose of green coffee bean extract. "Based on our results," he says, "taking multiple capsules of green coffee bean extract a day—while eating a low-fat, healthful diet and exercising regularly—appears to be a safe, effective, inexpensive way to lose weight."[36]

Questions Linger

The effectiveness (or lack thereof) of diet drugs is an issue with many variables and no simple answers. Studies have shown that drugs used in combination can be effective at helping people lose weight, and the same is true of clinical trials of the new diet drugs Belviq and Qsymia. The dietary supplement story is murkier, with some people claiming that the supplements are effective and others saying they are a waste of money. Whether people take drugs or supplements or not, there is one thing on which obesity experts and weight-loss specialists agree: Everyone can benefit from eating a healthier diet and being physically active.

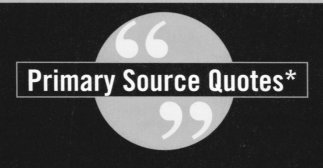

Primary Source Quotes*

How Effective Are Diet Drugs?

66 Simply taking pills, drinking shakes, applying creams, and all the other shortcuts that people search for will never be as effective in the long term as living and maintaining a better lifestyle. 99

—Vincent Bellonzi, *Health Recklessly Abandoned*. Garden City, NY: Morgan James, 2013, p. 12.

Bellonzi is a doctor of chiropractic medicine and a certified clinical nutritionist at the Austin Wellness Clinic in Austin, Texas.

66 The makers of weight-loss pills would like you to believe that their products will miraculously solve your weight problems. But keep in mind that even if you take a weight-loss pill, you still have to eat fewer calories than your body uses in order to lose weight. 99

—Mayo Clinic, "Over-the-Counter Weight-Loss Pills: Do They Work?," February 11, 2012. www.mayoclinic.com.

Mayo Clinic is a world-renowned health care facility headquartered in Rochester, Minnesota.

* Editor's Note: While the definition of a primary source can be narrowly or broadly defined, for the purposes of Compact Research, a primary source consists of: 1) results of original research presented by an organization or researcher; 2) eyewitness accounts of events, personal experience, or work experience; 3) first-person editorials offering pundits' opinions; 4) government officials presenting political plans and/or policies; 5) representatives of organizations presenting testimony or policy.

Primary Source Quotes

❝Shedding pounds takes effort and planning. There are simply no shortcuts.❞

—Andrew Weil, "Ask Dr. Weil: Should I Try Weight Loss Supplements?," *Prevention*, March 2013. www.prevention.com.

Weil is founder and director of the Arizona Center for Integrative Medicine and is a clinical professor of medicine at the University of Arizona.

❝Amphetamines have long been used as weight loss agents, although the wisdom of this use is controversial because weight loss is seldom sustained after the drug is stopped.❞

—Elaine A. Moore, *The Amphetamine Debate*. Jefferson, NC: McFarland, 2011, p. 28.

Moore is a medical technologist, laboratory consultant, and writer from Sedalia, Colorado.

❝Diet drugs often exert their weight loss effects only while the drug is being taken. This promotes 'yo-yo dieting,' which leads to more weight gain.❞

—Alliance for Natural Health, "FDA Advisory Panel Green-Lights Toxic Weight Loss Pill," February 28, 2012. www.anh-usa.org.

The Alliance for Natural Health is an organization that advocates a healthy diet and lifestyle and favors alternative medicine over drugs, surgery, and other conventional techniques.

❝Many people who take medications to lose weight regain the weight they lost when they stop taking the medication.❞

—Donald Hensrud, "Alli Weight-Loss Pill: Does It Work?," Mayo Clinic, February 11, 2012. www.mayoclinic.com.

Hensrud is a preventive medicine and nutrition specialist at Mayo Clinic in Rochester, Minnesota.

❝If you're hoping to lose weight, resist the lure of quick and easy solutions. What counts is a healthy lifestyle. Enjoy healthier foods and include physical activity in your daily routine.❞

—Katherine Zeratsky, "Are Vitamin B-12 Injections Helpful for Weight Loss?," Mayo Clinic, July 27, 2012. www.mayoclinic.com.

Zeratsky is a registered dietician at Mayo Clinic in Rochester, Minnesota.

....

❝Weight-loss medications lead to an average weight loss of about 10 pounds more than what you might lose with nondrug obesity treatments.❞

—National Institute of Diabetes and Digestive and Kidney Diseases (NIDDK), "Prescription Medications for the Treatment of Obesity," Weight Control Information Network, November 16, 2012. http://win.niddk.nih.gov.

The NIDDK conducts and supports medical research to improve people's health and quality of life.

....

How Effective Are Diet Drugs?

- During clinical trials of the diet drug Qnexa (now called Qsymia), patients taking the highest dose lost an average of **10.6 percent** of their body weight after a year, compared with the placebo group who lost **1.7 percent** of body weight.

- According to data from the North American Antiepileptic Drug Pregnancy Registry, for fetuses that are exposed to topiramate (one of the active ingredients in the diet drug Qsymia) during the first trimester of pregnancy there is a risk of being born with **cleft palate** that is twenty times higher than for infants who have not been exposed to the drug.

- In a Gallup poll conducted in November 2011 only **4 percent** of participants said they lost weight by taking diet drugs.

- The US Department of Health and Human Services says that FDA-approved diet drugs lead to an average weight loss that is only about **ten pounds** more than what the patient could achieve without the drugs.

- According to New York internal medicine specialist Steven Lamm, there are about ten **dietary supplements** on the market today that can prove to be useful in a weight-loss program.

- According to the National Institute of Diabetes and Digestive and Kidney Diseases, some antidepressant medications have been shown to work as **appetite suppressants**, but after six months patients often regain any weight they have lost even if they continue taking the medications.

New Diet Drug Proven Effective

In June 2012 the US Food and Drug Administration (FDA) approved the first new diet drug in thirteen years. Lorcaserin (trade name Belviq) had been tested in clinical trials and was found to be effective as part of a weight-loss regimen. This graph shows the results of a study in which participants who took lorcaserin achieved significantly better weight-loss results than those who took a placebo (dummy pills with no active medication).

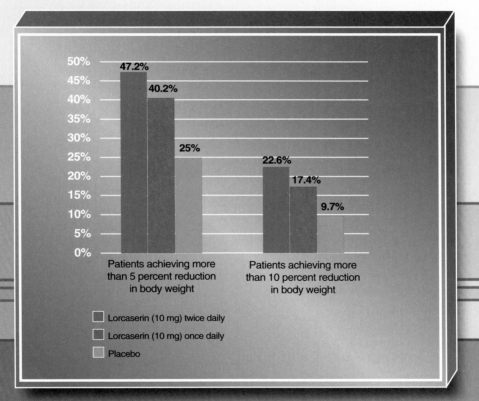

Source: Meredith C. Fidler et al., "A One-Year Randomized Trial of Lorcaserin for Weight Loss in Obese and Overweight Adults: The BLOSSOM Trial," *Journal of Clinical Endocrinology & Metabolism*, October 2011. http://jcem.endojournals.org.

• The June 2013 issue of the *UC Berkeley Wellness Letter* cites three studies in which people who took the diet drug Belviq for a year lost **3 percent to 4 percent** more weight (on average) than those taking a placebo.

Diet Drugs Not a Common Weight-Loss Strategy

In a Gallup poll conducted in November 2011 participants who said they had successfully lost weight were asked how they made it happen. As this chart shows, most people relied on changes in diet and/or exercise, with only 4 percent saying they took diet drugs.

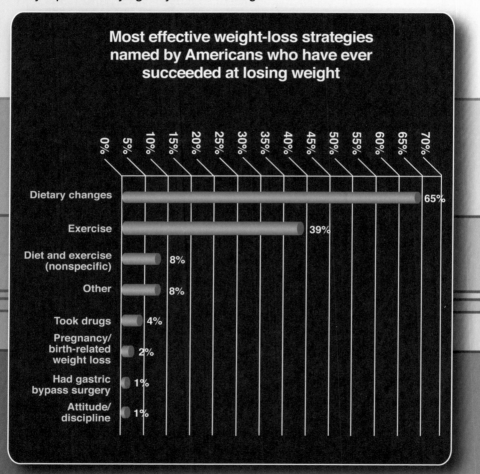

Most effective weight-loss strategies named by Americans who have ever succeeded at losing weight

Strategy	Percentage
Dietary changes	65%
Exercise	39%
Diet and exercise (nonspecific)	8%
Other	8%
Took drugs	4%
Pregnancy/birth-related weight loss	2%
Had gastric bypass surgery	1%
Attitude/discipline	1%

Source: Gallup, "To Lose Weight, Americans Rely More on Dieting than Exercise," November 28, 2011. www.gallup.com.

- According to physician and clinical researcher Judy Stone, studies have consistently revealed two disadvantages for people taking diet drugs: the drugs' efficacy tends to **plateau over time**, and the weight is regained when the drugs are stopped.

Negligible Effectiveness of OTC Diet Pills

Although people spend millions of dollars each year on diet drugs and other weight-loss aids, most of these products have not proved to be effective. Shown on this diagram are some of the most common over-the-counter (OTC) pills and supplements along with manufacturers' claims and the Mayo Clinic's perspective on effectiveness.

Product	Manufacturer Claim	Effectiveness
Alli (over-the-counter version of prescription drug called Xenical)	Decrease absorption of dietary fat	Effective, but weight loss is more modest than with Xenical
Bitter orange	Increases calories burned	Probably ineffective
Chitosan	Blocks absorption of dietary fat	Probably ineffective
Chromium	Decreases appetite and increases calories burned	Probably ineffective
Conjugated linoleic acid	Reduces body fat	Possibly effective
Green tea extract	Decreases appetite, increases calorie and fat metabolism	Insufficient evidence to evaluate
Guar gum	Blocks absorption of dietary fat and increases feeling of fullness	Possibly ineffective

Source: Mayo Clinic, "Over-the-Counter Weight-Loss Pills: Do They Work?," February 11, 2012. www.mayoclinic.com.

- The FDA states that the diet drug Belviq should be discontinued if someone fails to lose **5 percent** of his or her body weight after twelve weeks of treatment, as it is unlikely that continued treatment will be successful.

- According to Mayo Clinic dietician and nutritionist Katherine Zeratsky, there is no evidence that the popular nonprescription diet pill called Lipovarin promotes weight loss, and the product may actually pose **serious health risks**.

What Are the Health Risks of Diet Drugs?

66Some consumers believe that a product wouldn't be available if it wasn't proven to be safe, but unfortunately that's not the case.99

—Cynthia Sass, a registered dietician who holds master's degrees in both nutrition science and public health.

66Each year, women and men of all ages abuse diet pills and the result is a psychological and chemical addiction.99

—Seacliff Recovery Center, a full-service rehabilitation facility located in Huntington Beach, California.

With a mother, father, brother, and sister who were all physicians, it was only natural that Sarah Houston would also pursue a career in medicine, and she decided to do just that. The twenty-three-year-old medical student from England was known for her kindness and compassion. She was healthy, happy, popular with her friends, and a good student—but she also fought an ongoing battle: She was obsessed with her weight and struggled for years with eating disorders. Her family knew about her problem and that she had been seeing a psychiatrist for three years who was helping her overcome it. They had no idea, however, that she was taking a dangerous drug, DNP, in an attempt to lose weight, so they were shocked and grief-stricken in September 2012 when the drug killed her.

Banned but Not Gone

DNP's ability to speed up metabolism was first discovered in the United States during the 1930s. Even though it was an industrial chemical, it was initially hailed as a drug that could be of great benefit to people who wanted to lose weight—until it was linked to many dangerous and life-threatening health problems. DNP was banned in the United States in 1938, and also in the United Kingdom, and was rarely heard about for decades. Then, with the soaring growth of the Internet and availability of online drug sellers, DNP resurfaced. Websites often advertised it as a pesticide that was not for human consumption, although this was a ploy to avoid detection by law enforcement. Says police detective Kate Lonsdale: "By selling it in tablet form, they are knowing full well that it is going to be used for weight loss."[37]

Houston ordered her bottle of DNP from an online seller about eighteen months before her death, and she secretly began taking the pills. The night before she died, one of her roommates encouraged her to go to the hospital because her eyes had taken on a yellowish color, she was having trouble breathing, and she complained of feeling unbearably hot even after taking cool showers. Houston chose not to seek medical attention, saying that it was not unusual for her to have those symptoms and they would soon pass—and that was the last time anyone saw her alive. The next day another of her roommates found her dead at home, and an autopsy determined that Houston had died from a toxic reaction to DNP.

> " Websites often advertised [DNP] as a pesticide that was not for human consumption, although this was a deceptive ploy to avoid detection by law enforcement. "

At an inquest, coroner David Hinchliff stated that DNP was "entirely" responsible for her death, and he demanded a crackdown on online dealers who sell the dangerous chemical in capsule form. "The only motive for manufacturing a toxic substance as a slimming aid," Hinchliff said, "would be to profit from people who have the misfortune of having a condition such as Sarah's.

Anyone who professionally manufactures capsules to be taken as a drug has the intention of people using it as a drug. Sarah's death is a consequence of that."[38]

Toxic Supplements

Such tragic stories are not uncommon. Weight-loss supplements are widely available on the Internet, and consumers are often unaware that they are not subject to the same oversight by the FDA as drugs are. Pieter A. Cohen, an internist at Cambridge Health Alliance and an assistant professor of medicine at Harvard Medical School, cites a public opinion survey in which the majority of respondents believed that dietary supplements were approved by a government agency. Two-thirds of respondents were under the impression that the government requires labels on supplements to include warnings about their potential side effects and dangers. Neither of these assumptions is correct.

As surprising as it may be, health care professionals have also proved to be uninformed about the issue. Surveys have shown that many physicians mistakenly believe that dietary supplements require FDA approval and, says Cohen, "the majority did not know that adverse events suspected to have been caused by supplements should be reported to the FDA."[39]

> " Many supplements are believed to be made in developing countries such as Brazil and China where quality control measures are lax or nonexistent. "

Companies that manufacture dietary supplements, including those that are labeled as weight-loss aids, are not bound by federal guidelines for the purity, effectiveness, quality, and safety of their products. Dozens of dietary supplements have been found to contain a wide variety of substances such as amphetamines, toxic plant material, heavy metals, experimental compounds, and even drugs that were previously rejected by the FDA because of safety concerns. Michael Levy, director of the FDA's Division of New Drugs and Labeling Compliance, explains: "We've found other weight-loss products marketed as supplements that contain dangerous concoctions of hidden ingredients including seizure medications, blood pressure medications, and other drugs not approved in the U.S."[40]

A major problem with online ordering of weight-loss supplements is that so much about them is unknown. For instance, consumers usually have no way of knowing who the manufacturers are or in what country the products were made. Many supplements are believed to be made in developing countries such as Brazil and China where quality control measures are lax or nonexistent.

This was found to be the case with weight-loss supplements known as StarCaps, which are made in Peru and sold on the Internet and in vitamin/nutrition stores in the United States. They were promoted as all-natural dietary supplements that contained papaya, but an FDA investigation found that there was much more to them than that. The supplements also contained a potent pharmaceutical drug called bumetanide, which is used to reduce swelling and fluid retention caused by various medical problems, as well as to treat high blood pressure. Says Levy, "We don't think consumers should be using these products."[41]

The Ugly Side of Fat Blockers

People who have used the diet drug called orlistat, which is available with a doctor's prescription as Xenical and over the counter as Alli, are undoubtedly very familiar with the drug's unpleasant and sometimes messy side effects. There are potential risks associated with these drugs, however, that go far beyond runny stools and oily spotting. An August 2009 article in *Consumer Reports* tells of several thousand adverse events related to the drug that were reported to the FDA beginning in January 2007, including rectal bleeding and kidney, liver, and thyroid problems. Charles Bennett, director of the Research on Adverse Drug Events and Reports (RADAR) group, says that "this safety concern is heightened when one considers that only an estimated 1 percent to 10 percent of all adverse events that occur are ever reported to the FDA."[42]

A more recent study was published in December 2012 by University of Rhode Island professor Bingfang Yan, a pharmacologist who is well known for his discoveries of dangerous drug interactions. During his study, Yan found that orlistat interferes with a major detoxification enzyme, and this may lead to severe toxicity of internal organs such as the liver or kidneys. "Since it has been available over-the-counter," says

> **During his study, Yan found that orlistat interferes with a major detoxification enzyme, and this may lead to severe toxicity of internal organs such as the liver or kidneys.**

Yan, "there has been a drastic increase of toxicity among patients using the drug. It has been linked to severe liver failure, acute pancreatic failure, and acute renal (kidney) failure." According to Yan, it is generally assumed that orlistat remains in the intestine and that the body does not absorb it, but this has proved to be a flawed theory. "Orlistat is reportedly absorbed," he says, "and certainly internal organs such as the liver and kidney are exposed to this drug upon absorption."[43]

In addition to toxicity problems, Yan's study uncovered another problem with orlistat: when it is used by people who take certain medications, it interferes with the drugs' ability to work properly. This is true of drugs that are prescribed to treat people with cancer, as Yan explains: "This study shows that orlistat profoundly alters the therapeutic potential of the anticancer drugs . . . it weakens their effectiveness."[44]

Potent and Unsafe

During the 1990s people who wanted to slim down were able to buy weight-loss supplements that contained ephedra, a natural stimulant from a shrub of the same name that is native to China. Like all stimulants, ephedra speeds up the heart rate and boosts metabolism, which is why it helps promote weight loss. In 2004 the FDA banned the use of ephedra in dietary supplements after receiving hundreds of reports of serious and life-threatening problems including heart attacks and seizures, and more than a hundred deaths. The US Department of Health and Human Services explains: "After a careful review of the available evidence about the risks and benefits of ephedra in supplements, the FDA found that these supplements present an unreasonable risk of illness or injury to consumers. The data showed . . . that the substance raises blood pressure and stresses the heart. The increased risk of heart problems and strokes negates any benefits of weight loss."[45]

Although ephedra may not be used in dietary supplements sold in the United States, its synthetic cousin, ephedrine, is still used in cold and allergy medications. It is not approved as a diet drug, but because it speeds up metabolism, some people use it for weight loss. One woman from the United Kingdom who used ephedrine in this way is Michelle Rumsey. After combing through online forums to get tips about weight-loss drugs, she learned about how effective ephedrine is for people who wanted to lose weight. So, she ordered some ephedrine pills from an online seller in Canada.

Rumsey started taking two ephedrine tablets per day, and, as she had hoped, the pounds started melting away. Yet she felt herself becoming addicted to the drug, as she explains: "The pills kept my appetite down and I was convinced that if I stopped taking them, the weight would pile back on." She continued taking the pills for the next two years and then started having strange side effects. "I felt light-headed," she says. "The room was blurred and my heart was racing. After ten minutes, my heart rate went back to normal, but I was terrified. I was sure the pills were to blame and threw them in the [trash] bin."[46] One incident was particularly frightening for Rumsey. She was on a bike ride with her boyfriend when she suddenly started having chest pains. Over the next few weeks she noticed herself becoming more out of breath, and within a month she found it "hard to walk up half a flight of stairs without gasping for air."[47]

> **The greatest dangers are with dietary supplements because so much about them is unknown, including where they are manufactured and what they contain.**

Rumsey was examined by a heart and lung specialist who gave her devastating news: The ephedrine had constricted the vessels in her lungs, which put immense pressure on her heart. This led to a condition known as pulmonary hypertension, or high blood pressure in the arteries of the lungs that can lead to heart and lung failure. At the time of her diagnosis, Rumsey was told that she had a life expectancy of only ten more years. "I couldn't stop crying when the doctor told me what was wrong," she says. She realizes that the damage has been done and there is no cure for her condition. "I'm angry and depressed that I have effectively been handed a death sentence," she says. "It never occurred to me that these pills could be so dangerous."[48]

Worth the Risk?

Although they may not be aware of it, people who use diet drugs and weight-loss supplements are taking a risk with their health. The greatest dangers are with dietary supplements because so much about them is unknown, including where they are manufactured and what they contain. But even FDA-approved drugs can be risky, as was shown in studies of orlistat. People who want to lose weight may still choose to use diet drugs, but it is important that they fully understand not only the benefits but also the potential risks. Only then can they make an informed decision about whether taking a chance with their health is worth it.

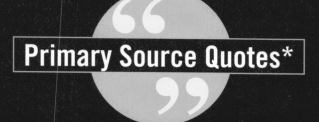

What Are the Health Risks of Diet Drugs?

❝A number of weight-loss pills are available at your local drugstore, supermarket or health food store. Even more options are available online. Most haven't been proved effective, and some may be downright dangerous.❞

—Mayo Clinic, "Over-the-Counter Weight-Loss Pills: Do They Work?," February 11, 2012. www.mayoclinic.com.

Mayo Clinic is a world-renowned health care facility headquartered in Rochester, Minnesota.

....

❝In the last few years, FDA has discovered hundreds of dietary supplements containing drugs or other chemicals, often in products for weight loss and body-building. . . . They could cause serious side effects or interact in dangerous ways with medicines or other supplements you're taking.❞

—Federal Trade Commission (FTC), "Weighing the Claims in Diet Ads," July 2012. www.consumer.ftc.gov.

The FTC is a government agency that exists to protect American consumers from fraud and unfair business practices and to ensure fair competition.

....

* Editor's Note: While the definition of a primary source can be narrowly or broadly defined, for the purposes of Compact Research, a primary source consists of: 1) results of original research presented by an organization or researcher; 2) eyewitness accounts of events, personal experience, or work experience; 3) first-person editorials offering pundits' opinions; 4) government officials presenting political plans and/or policies; 5) representatives of organizations presenting testimony or policy.

66 Drugs may give apparent results because you lose weight, but this is not without the price of side effects and perhaps even permanent damage to your body. 99

—Vincent Bellonzi, *Health Recklessly Abandoned*. Garden City, NY: Morgan James, 2013, p. 12.

Bellonzi is a doctor of chiropractic medicine and a certified clinical nutritionist at the Austin Wellness Clinic in Austin, Texas.

66 For some reason, FDA thinks the benefits of taking an expensive pill to lose a tiny bit of weight outweigh the crippling headaches, mental problems, and depression. 99

—Alliance for Natural Health, "A New Diet Pill Hits the Market," July 3, 2012. www.anh-usa.org.

The Alliance for Natural Health is an organization that advocates a healthy diet and lifestyle and favors alternative medicine over drugs, surgery, and other conventional techniques.

66 As a class, weight loss supplements are ineffective, and several have proven to be dangerous. Many are based on stimulants that can elevate blood pressure and cause irregular heartbeat, anxiety, and insomnia. 99

—Andrew Weil, "Ask Dr. Weil: Should I Try Weight Loss Supplements?," *Prevention*, March 2013. www.prevention.com.

Weil is founder and director of the Arizona Center for Integrative Medicine and is a clinical professor of medicine at the University of Arizona.

66 Although most side effects of prescription medications for obesity are mild, serious complications have been reported. 99

—National Institute of Diabetes and Digestive and Kidney Diseases (NIDDK), "Prescription Medications for the Treatment of Obesity," Weight Control Information Network, November 16, 2012. http://win.niddk.nih.gov.

The NIDDK conducts and supports medical research to improve people's health and quality of life.

❝Diet pills contain such chemicals as laxatives, caffeine and ephedrine, and these additives can cause serious problems and permanent damage.❞

—Elements Behavioral Health, "Diet Pill Addiction: It Isn't Worth the Weight," July 5, 2011. www.treatmentcenters.net.

Elements Behavioral Health, which is headquartered in Long Beach, California, offers specialized addiction treatment programs at a number of locations.

....

❝There's no evidence that Lipovarin—a popular, non-prescription diet pill—promotes weight loss. In fact, this product may actually pose serious health risks.❞

—Katherine Zeratsky, "Lipovarin: An Effective Weight-Loss Supplement?," Mayo Clinic, December 11, 2012. www.mayoclinic.com.

Zeratsky is a registered dietician at Mayo Clinic in Rochester, Minnesota.

....

Facts and Illustrations

What Are the Health Risks of Diet Drugs?

- Once a common ingredient in weight-loss supplements, the stimulant ephedra was banned in 2004 after causing more than sixteen thousand adverse health events, including cases of **stroke and death**.

- According to a 2011 report published in the *Journal of Medical Toxicology*, sixty-two deaths have been reported in medical literature as the result of the chemical **dinitrophenol (DNP)** being used as a diet drug.

- In 2010 and 2011, clinical trials with the diet drug Belviq showed that the most common adverse effects were **headache, dizziness, fatigue, nausea, dry mouth, and constipation**.

- According to the National Institute of Diabetes and Digestive and Kidney Diseases, **amphetamines** are appetite suppressants, but they are not recommended for use in treating obesity due to their strong potential for abuse and dependence.

- The FDA states that manufacturers of both Belviq and Qsymia (diet drugs approved in 2012) will be required to perform long-term clinical trials to examine the drugs' effects on the risk for **heart attacks and stroke**.

Most Dieters Willing to Risk Some Drug Side Effects

During a national health care survey conducted in August 2010, participants were asked what side effects they would be willing to accept while taking diet drugs or supplements to reach their weight-loss goal. As this graph shows, the level of side effects that most people were willing to accept was proportional to how overweight they were.

Participants Willing to Risk . . .

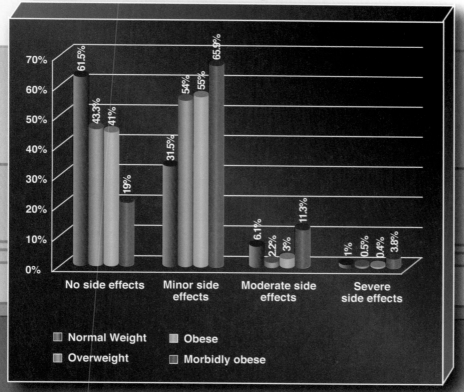

Source: Thomson Reuters, "National Survey of Healthcare Consumers: Weight Loss," August 2010. www.factsforhealthcare.com.

- The FDA states that the diet drug Qsymia carries a high risk for **birth defects** (cleft lip and palate) in infants exposed to it during the first trimester of pregnancy.

Risky Diet Drugs Pulled by FDA

All prescription diet drugs must be approved by the FDA before they can be used by the public. Approval decisions are based on safety and effectiveness. Some drugs never make it to market. Some are pulled from the market after receiving approval. This chart shows five diet drugs that have been rejected or withdrawn since 1997 and the reasons why.

Rejected or withdrawn weight-loss drugs

Drug Name	Manufacturer	Year Pulled	Why
Contrave (bupropion, naltrexone)	Orexigen	2011	Elevated heart rate, blood pressure
Meridia (sibutramine)	Abbott	2010	Increased risk of heart attack, stroke
Qnexa (phentermine, topiramate)	Vivus	2010	Increased heart rate, possible birth defects
Lorqess (lorcaserin*)	Arena	2010	Breast cancer in lab animals
Acomplia (rimonabant)	Sanofi-Aventis	2007	Depression, suicidal thoughts

* In 2012 the FDA approved lorcaserin under a new trade name (Belviq), and approved Qnexa under the new name of Qsymia.

Source: Kathleen Doheny, "The Real Dangers of Weight-Loss Drugs," *Consumers Digest*, May 2011. www.consumersdigest.com.

- According to Andrew Weil, founder and director of the Arizona Center for Integrative Medicine and clinical professor of medicine at the University of Arizona, weight-loss supplements often contain stimulant drugs that can **elevate blood pressure and cause irregular heartbeat, anxiety, and insomnia.**

- The National Institutes of Health states that the diet drug Topiramate causes a fairly high incidence of **confusion, memory loss, and concentration problems.**

Risks of the Chinese Diet Drug Pai You Guo

In 2009 the FDA announced that an over-the-counter diet supplement made in China called Pai You Guo contained ingredients that were not safe, so the drug was to be withdrawn from the market. But a study published in 2011 found that a cluster of women from Massachusetts were still using the drug and many had experienced side effects from it. Some of the prevalent effects are shown here.

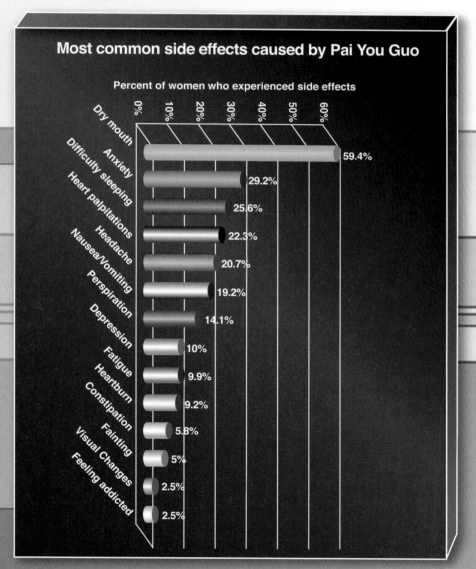

Most common side effects caused by Pai You Guo

Percent of women who experienced side effects

Side effect	Percent
Dry mouth	59.4%
Anxiety	29.2%
Difficulty sleeping	25.6%
Heart palpitations	22.3%
Headache	20.7%
Nausea/Vomiting	19.2%
Perspiration	14.1%
Depression	10%
Fatigue	9.9%
Heartburn	9.2%
Constipation	5.8%
Fainting	5%
Visual Changes	2.5%
Feeling addicted	2.5%

Source: Pieter A. Cohen, Carly Benner, and Danny McCormick, "Use of a Pharmaceutically Adulterated Dietary Supplement, Pai You Guo, Among Brazilian-Born Women in the United States," *Journal of General Internal Medicine*, 2011. www.ncbi.nim.nih.gov.

How Big a Problem Is Diet-Drug Fraud?

66American consumers lose billions of dollars each year to health fraud schemes. Worse than losing your money, you could lose your health.99

—US Food and Drug Administration, a federal agency that is responsible for protecting the public health by assuring the safety and effectiveness of America's food supply, human and veterinary drugs, and other products.

66Anything advertised as a 'miracle cure' is likely to be a scam—no matter how clever the marketing may be.99

—Andrew Weil, founder and director of the Arizona Center for Integrative Medicine and a clinical professor of medicine at the University of Arizona.

Many people who have searched the web for information on the latest diets have run across intriguing articles about weight-loss products made from acai berries. These are reddish-purple fruits that are about an inch (2.54 cm) long and come from the acai palm tree, which is native to the Amazon rain forest. Sometimes called "super foods," acai berries are nutritious and contain numerous beneficial substances. For instance, they are high in antioxidants, and are believed to help reduce cholesterol levels and naturally increase energy. Despite the many benefits, there is no evidence that supplements made with acai berries promote rapid weight loss—yet that is what a number of companies have claimed on their websites.

On some of these sites are striking headlines such as, "Acai Berry

Diet Exposed: Miracle Diet or Scam?" The text beneath the headline is presented as though it is a testimonial by a news reporter, one of whom is "News 6 health and diet reporter named Julia Millar." The article explains that after seeing innumerable ads for acai berry supplements, Millar decided to investigate to see if the claims were valid, and in doing so she "volunteered to be the guinea pig."[49] She placed an order for a four-week supply of acai berry supplements, and when the package arrived she started putting the program to a test. She kept people updated about her progress on the weight-loss program by commenting periodically on the website.

At the end of four weeks Millar said she was stunned to have lost 25 pounds (11.34 kg). She also said that her energy levels were higher and she was sleeping better at night, which left her feeling more rested in the morning. On the "Results" section of the site, a post from Millar states: "I couldn't be any happier with the results. I lost 25 lbs in 4 weeks, no special diet, no intense exercise." She went on to encourage others to see for themselves how fabulous the acai berry weight-loss program was, saying, "Like us, here at News 6, you might be a little doubtful about the effects of this diet, but you need to try it for yourself; the results are real."[50]

> There is no evidence that supplements made with acai berries can promote rapid weight loss—yet that is what a number of companies have promoted on their websites.

Clamping Down

But the results were not "real" at all; the whole campaign was found to be phony. There was no reporter named Julia Millar, and the website information was nothing more than advertising designed to look like a news story. According to Donald Vladeck, director of the Federal Trade Commission (FTC) Bureau of Consumer Protection, the same is true of all sites of this nature, as he explains: "Almost everything about these sites is fake. The weight loss results, the so-called investigations, the reporters, the consumer testimonials, and the attempt to portray an objective, journalistic endeavor."[51]

In April 2011 the FTC announced that it was seeking to permanently stop the misleading acai berry campaign and asked the courts to freeze the assets of ten operations that were behind it. In court documents the FTC stated that the defendants posted attention-grabbing ads on search engines and high-volume websites for the purpose of intentionally driving traffic to the fake news sites. The ultimate goal, according to the FTC, was for consumers to be sold on the acai berry weight-loss program based on testimonials, which would compel them to visit the sites where the products were sold. The FTC explains: "The sites supposedly report on the effectiveness of acai berry dietary supplements to help people with dramatic weight loss. But the reporters making big weight-loss claims are phony, made up by marketers selling supplements. And in some cases, once you sign up, you might end up enrolled in an expensive 'free trial.'"[52]

> " In April 2011 the FTC announced that it was seeking to permanently stop the misleading acai berry campaign and asked the courts to freeze the assets of ten operations that were behind it. "

By the time the FTC went after ten of the bogus operations, it had received numerous complaints from people who had been deceived by the promises in the fake campaign. The agency discovered that the defendants received commissions when consumers bought the products or signed up for "free trials" on the websites. Also according to the FTC, the defendants paid more than $10 million to run the fraudulent campaign and "have likely received well in excess of that amount in ill-gotten commissions."[53]

Connecticut Huckster

One weight-loss scammer the FTC claims cheated people out of an estimated $25 million is Boris Mizhen, a man from Guilford, Connecticut. According to the FTC, Mizhen owns several companies: LeanSpa and NutraSlim in the United States, and NutraSlim UK, which is based in the United Kingdom. On television commercials, actors posing as news reporters gushed about how they (like the fabricated reporter Julia Millar) had "lost up to 25 pounds in a month without any special diet or exercise!"[54] Also promised was a no-cost, risk-free trial, and satisfaction was 100 percent guaranteed.

A young woman named Melissa who worked as an orthodontic assistant was somewhat interested in the offer. She was not overweight but thought that maybe the initial thirty-day supply of acai berry supplements would enable her to lose about five pounds. She wondered, "What would a free trial hurt?"[55] and she placed her order.

Melissa suspected that she had been scammed when shortly after receiving her "free trial" products in the mail, she saw a charge on her credit card for $79.99. "So it wasn't free," says Melissa, "if they're charging you $80. Then they turned around and said they were charging $80 for the next shipment. Well, the next shipment should not have gone out for 30 days."[56] Melissa did not have a good feeling about the company, so she returned the acai berry capsules and followed up by calling the company on the telephone. When a credit did not appear on her credit card she kept after the company, as well as reporting it to the Better Business Bureau. According to the FTC, that sort of aggressive follow-through is not common; many people become so frustrated they just give up and do not pursue it when money is owed to them. Scammers count on this, and it is a big part of how they make so much money.

By the time the FTC and the Connecticut attorney general stepped in, more than eleven hundred complaints had been filed against Mizhen's companies in less than a year. Melissa was finally credited for the $79.99—but only because she complained. "I was adamant about it," she says. "It was wrong and I didn't want it happening to other people. I'm strong enough to fight it. I didn't care how long it took me."[57]

Fakery Abounds

The FTC is charged with a monumental job: protecting American consumers by preventing fraud, deception, and unfair business practices in the marketplace. Scammers promote their products in numerous ways, including through newspaper and magazine advertising, television infomercials, and the Internet. The FDA writes: "You can find health fraud scams in retail stores and on countless websites, in popup ads and spam, and on social media sites like Facebook and Twitter."[58]

Among the FTC's tasks are to conduct regular surveys of Americans who have been victims of fraud and to publish the results on the FTC website. For purposes of the survey, the agency considers weight-loss products to include nonprescription (over-the-counter) drugs, dietary supplements, skin patches, creams, wraps, and weight-loss earrings. The FTC determines which weight-loss products are fraudulent based on whether they are being promoted as enabling consumers to easily lose a substantial amount of weight or to lose the weight without diet or exercise. "However," says the FTC, "when consumers purchased and used the product, they lost less than half of the weight they had expected to lose, if they lost any weight at all."[59]

> " Scammers promote their products in numerous ways, including through newspaper and magazine advertising, television infomercials, and the Internet. "

In April 2013 the FTC published a survey it conducted in 2012. Researchers found that in 2011 more consumers in the United States were victims of fraudulent weight-loss-product scams than of any other type of fraud. The report states that an estimated 7.6 million incidents of weight-loss fraud occurred during the year, meaning that an estimated 5.1 million American adults (2.1 percent of consumers) purchased and used fraudulent weight-loss products. These numbers were significantly higher than in other types of fraud such as fraudulent prize promotions, being billed for a buyers' club membership that one did not agree to purchase, being billed for Internet services that one did not agree to purchase, and work-at-home programs.

The FTC is sometimes criticized because of all the weight-loss-drug scams that exist and the fact that millions of consumers are victims of these scams each year. But the agency's resources are limited, and its investigators must sift through thousands of products and advertisements. This is a daunting task, as Steven Novella explains: "To its credit, the FTC has been going after false advertising of supplements, but there are so many products and companies you can simply hide in the herd. Many of the cases the FTC goes after lied in their advertising or used deceptive practices other than just making up claims for random ingredients."[60]

The Questionable HCG

In December 2011 the FDA and FTC launched a joint effort to stop companies from marketing over-the-counter products known as human chorionic gonadotropin, or HCG. This is a hormone that is found in the urine of pregnant women. It is made by cells that form in the placenta, which nourishes the egg after it has been fertilized. As a prescription medication, HCG is used to treat certain other medical conditions, including infertility. It has not, however, been approved for over-the-counter use, nor is there any proof that it can help people lose weight. Companies marketing over-the-counter HCG weight-loss products labeled as "homeopathic" were sent warning letters from the FTC and FDA. The letters cautioned that the companies were violating federal law by selling the unapproved drugs and by making unsupported claims for their products. According to the US Department of Health and Human Services Office on Women's Health, HCG products touted as weight-loss aids are sold online and in stores, despite the absence of proof that they are effective.

Sellers typically recommended that the products be taken along with an extremely low-calorie diet—as low as five hundred calories per day. The website for one seller claimed that people who take Original HCG Drops could lose up to thirty pounds in thirty to forty days. The Office on Women's Health writes: "The company also claims that HCG 'tells the body to release abnormal fat' and 'hold on to lean muscle. All this is designed to establish a new body weight and reset your metabolism.'"[61]

> " The FTC is sometimes criticized because of all the weight-loss-drug scams that exist and the fact that millions of consumers are victims of these scams each year. "

In a statement supporting the joint FDA-FTC effort to get HCG off the market, dietician and nutritionist Samantha Heller says: "The HCG diet is a typical fad diet that preys on people's desperation for fast weight loss. Not only is it dangerous for people to consume only 500 calories a day over time but the safety and efficacy of taking HCG for weight loss has not been established. A near starvation diet can result in emotional, psychological and physiological damage."[62]

Once the targeted companies receive their warning letters, they have fifteen days to notify the FDA of measures they have taken or will take to correct the violations. If they fail to respond, the companies may face enforcement action, possible legal penalties, and/or criminal prosecution. In addition to targeting companies that sell HCG, the FDA has issued public advisories to inform consumers that they should stop using the product right away.

A Formidable Challenge

Protecting consumers from fraud is an enormously challenging task. Research shows that millions of Americans are victimized by fraudulent claims each year, and the most prevalent type of fraud is weight-loss scams. The FDA and FTC do their best to keep control of fraudulent acts, but it is impossible to completely stop them. As time goes by, perhaps new ways of monitoring and addressing fraud will be developed. Until then, consumers remain at risk of being scammed.

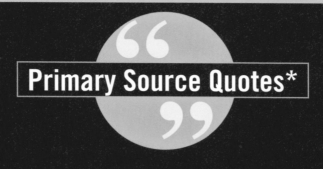

Primary Source Quotes*

How Big a Problem Is Diet-Drug Fraud?

66 With drugs, the standards are rigorous: Any drug product that is approved for sale must be shown to be equivalent to the product studied in the clinical trials that established its efficacy.... The same can't be said for supplements. 99

—Scott Gavura, "What's Really in Your Supplement?," (blog), Science-Based Pharmacy, May 3, 2013. http://sciencebasedpharmacy.wordpress.com.

Gavura is a pharmacist from Ontario, Canada.

66 Mainstream media like to portray the world of nutritional supplements as the Wild West, with nothing to protect the unwary consumer.... The charge is false. Supplements and supplement manufacturing are highly regulated. 99

—Alliance for Natural Health, "Supplement Safety: What You Need to Know About ConsumerLab.com—and More," June 5, 2012. www.anh-usa.org.

The Alliance for Natural Health is an organization that advocates a healthy diet and lifestyle and favors alternative medicine over drugs, surgery, and other conventional techniques.

Bracketed quotes indicate conflicting positions.

* Editor's Note: While the definition of a primary source can be narrowly or broadly defined, for the purposes of Compact Research, a primary source consists of: 1) results of original research presented by an organization or researcher; 2) eyewitness accounts of events, personal experience, or work experience; 3) first-person editorials offering pundits' opinions; 4) government officials presenting political plans and/or policies; 5) representatives of organizations presenting testimony or policy.

❝There really is no meaningful difference, in my opinion, between the modern supplement industry and the patent medicine hucksters of the 19th and early 20th centuries. The marketing hype is similar, as is the ploy of mixing in some actual drugs.❞

—Steven Novella, "You Got Drugs in My Weight Loss Supplement," *NeuroLogica* (blog), October 14, 2010. http://theness.com.

Novella is a clinical neurologist at Yale University School of Medicine.

....

❝Bottom line: Steer clear of weight-loss products that make unproven claims.❞

—Katherine Zeratsky, "Can Cortisol Blockers Such as CortiSlim Help Me Lose Weight?," Mayo Clinic, February 25, 2012. www.mayoclinic.com.

Zeratsky is a registered dietician at Mayo Clinic in Rochester, Minnesota.

....

❝Health fraud involves selling drugs, devices, foods or cosmetics that have not been proven effective. At best, these scams don't work. At worst, they're dangerous.❞

—National Institutes of Health, "Health Fraud," May 6, 2013. www.nlm.nih.gov.

The National Institutes of Health is the United States' leading medical research agency.

....

❝At best, products promising lightning-fast weight loss are a scam. At worst, they can ruin your health.❞

—Federal Trade Commission (FTC), "Weighing the Claims in Diet Ads," July 2012. www.consumer.ftc.gov.

The FTC is a government agency that exists to protect American consumers from fraud and unfair business practices and ensure fair competition.

....

66 People looking to lose weight will do almost anything to achieve fast weight loss. However, all too often these diets and pills turn out to be another scam. 99

—Nutrition Awareness and Conference Association of America (NACAA), "Raspberry Ultra Drops Another Weight Loss Scam," February 28, 2013. http://nacaa.net.

The NACAA seeks to spread awareness of healthy ways to lose weight and maintain physical fitness.

66 The label of a dietary supplement product is required to be truthful and not misleading. If the label does not meet this requirement, FDA may remove the product from the marketplace or take other appropriate action. 99

—Office of Dietary Supplements, "Background Information: Dietary Supplements," June 24, 2011. http://ods.od.nih.gov.

An agency of the National Institutes of Health, the Office of Dietary Supplements seeks to strengthen knowledge and understanding of dietary supplements.

Facts and Illustrations

How Big a Problem Is Diet-Drug Fraud?

- A survey by the Federal Trade Commission (FTC) that was published in 2013 revealed that more than one in ten American adults (about 26.5 million) were victims of fraud in 2011, and the most common type was **weight-loss-product fraud**.

- According to Yale University clinical neurologist Steven Novella, many of the claims the FTC pursues have involved **lying in advertising** or the use of **deceptive practices**.

- In 2012 the FTC sued Central Coast Neutraceuticals for deceptive advertising, fraudulent free trial offers, phony endorsements, and unfair billing, regarding their acai berry supplements, colon cleansers, and other such weight-loss products. The company was ordered to pay more than **$1.5 million for customer refunds**.

- According to Cleveland Clinic cardiologist Steven Nissen, the ability of the FDA to police the safety of supplements is limited by the scope of the industry; estimates of the number of supplements on the market range from **forty thousand to seventy-five thousand**.

- In a survey by the FTC that was published in 2013, Hispanics were found to be **60 percent** more likely to be victims of fraudulent weight-loss products than non-Hispanic whites.

Weight-Loss Scams Are the Most Common Type of Consumer Fraud

In the United States, the federal agency that is responsible for monitoring consumer fraud is the Federal Trade Commission and one of its responsibilities is conducting surveys to assess consumer experiences with fraud. The most recent survey, published in April 2013, found that between 22.4 million and 28.7 million American adults were victims of one or more types of fraud, with the most common type involving fraudulent weight-loss products.

American adults who were victims of fraud, 2011

Type of Fraud	Average Number of Victims (in millions)
Weight-loss products	5.1
Prize promotions	2.4
Unauthorized billing—buyers' clubs	1.9
Unauthorized billing—Internet services	1.9
Work-at-home-programs	1.8
Credit repair	1.7
Debt relief	1.5
Credit card insurance	1.3
Business opportunities	1.1
Mortgage relief	0.8
Advance-fee loans	0.7
Pyramid schemes	0.7
Government job offers	0.5
Counterfeit-check scams	0.4
Grant scams	0.2

Source: Keith B. Anderson, "Consumer Fraud in the United States, 2011: The Third FTC Survey," Federal Trade Commission, April 2013. www.ftc.gov.

- According to the FDA, any consumer can spot a fraudulent product by looking for **keywords** such as, "It works overnight," "revolutionary scientific breakthrough," "miracle cure," or "alternative to drugs or surgery."

Exaggerated Claims

The FDA regularly issues publications to warn people about scams involving foods or over-the-counter dietary products, including weight-loss supplements. Shown here are some of the potential warning signs of scams, including products that are potentially harmful because they contain unsafe ingredients.

Potential Warning Signs of Fraud

Unrealistic promises, such as "Melt your fat away!" or "Diet and exercise not required!"

Extreme claims, such as "Quick and effective" or "Totally safe"

Promises of quick action, such as "Lose 10 pounds in one week"

Use of the words "guaranteed" or "scientific breakthrough"

Labeled or marketed in a foreign language

Marketed through mass e-mails

Marketed as an herbal alternative to an FDA-approved drug, or as having effects similar to prescription drugs

Source: Food and Drug Administration, "Beware of Fraudulent Weight-Loss 'Dietary Supplements,'" March 15, 2011. www.fda.gov.

- In 2012 the British pharmaceutical company GlaxoSmithKline pleaded guilty and agreed to pay **$3 billion** in fraud settlements for false advertising on many of its pharmaceutical products, including the antidepressant Wellbutrin, which the company claimed aided in weight loss.

- The National Institutes of Health states that most victims of health-related scams are over the age of **sixty-five**.

- In 2011 US authorities issued a warning about **fake weight-loss products** being marketed as legitimate FDA-approved substances.

- According to Yale University clinical neurologist Steven Novella, as long as supplement manufacturers do not make claims about **preventing** or **curing disease**, it is difficult for the FDA to go after them for fraud.

- In a March 2013 report on health-fraud scams, the FDA states that its laboratories have found more than one hundred weight-loss products that are being **illegally marketed** as dietary substances.

Key People and Advocacy Groups

Alliance for Natural Health: An advocacy organization that promotes healthy diet and lifestyle and favors alternative medicine over drugs, surgery, and other conventional techniques.

Michael Anchors: An obesity specialist from Gaithersburg, Maryland, who created a diet-drug combo known as phen-Pro, which contains the appetite-suppressant drug phentermine and the antidepressant Prozac.

Louis Aronne: An internationally recognized obesity specialist who is director of the Comprehensive Weight Control Program at New York–Presbyterian Hospital/Weill Cornell Medical Center.

Michael Cowley: Former chief scientific officer of the pharmaceutical company Orexigen Therapeutics and inventor of the weight-loss drug Contrave.

Federal Trade Commission (FTC): A government agency that exists to protect American consumers from fraud and unfair business practices and to ensure fair competition.

Michael S. Lauer: One of only two members of a twenty-two-member FDA panel who voted against approving the diet drug Qnexa.

Joseph A. Mercola: An alternative-medicine physician who is critical of standard medical practices, advocates natural health solutions and dietary supplements, and who has been warned on several occasions by the FDA about making false claims regarding his products' ability to detect, prevent, and treat disease.

Thomas Najarian: A physician from Los Osos, California, who invented the diet drug Qnexa, which was later renamed Qsymia.

Richard Siegel: A well-known weight-loss expert who codirects the Diabetes Center at Tufts Medical Center in Boston and is a staff endocrinologist at the facility's Weight and Wellness Center.

Steven Smith: An obesity expert and scientific director of Florida Hospital's Translational Research Institute for Metabolism and Diabetes.

Maurice L. Tainter, Windsor C. Cutting, and A.B. Stockton: Stanford University physicians who in the 1930s found that the industrial chemical dinitrophenol (DNP) could speed up metabolism and promote weight loss; later they discovered that the drug had dangerous side effects.

US Food and Drug Administration (FDA): A federal agency that is charged with protecting the public health by assuring the safety and effectiveness of America's food supply, human and veterinary drugs, and other products.

Michael Weintraub: A pharmacologist from the University of Rochester in Rochester, New York, who came up with the idea of combining two diet drugs to make one that was more effective; the result was the infamous fen-phen combination, which proved to be successful but was later determined to carry a number of health risks.

Bingfang Yan: A University of Rhode Island professor and pharmacologist who is well known for his discoveries of dangerous drug interactions, which he chronicled in a book called *Encyclopedia of Drug Metabolism and Interactions*.

Chronology

1885
Japanese pharmacologist Nagayoshi Nagai is the first to identify and extract the stimulant ephedrine from the ephedra shrub.

1887
Working in a laboratory at the University of Berlin, Romanian chemist Lazăr Edeleanu becomes the first person to synthesize amphetamine.

1971
The FDA classifies amphetamines as Schedule II drugs, meaning they are recognized as having therapeutic value but also have a high potential for abuse and addiction. Doctors are urged to use caution when prescribing the drugs for their patients who want to lose weight.

1885   **1930**   **1970**

1938
Congress passes the Federal Food, Drug, and Cosmetic Act to replace the Federal Food and Drugs Act and establishes the Food and Drug Administration (FDA) to enforce the new law.

1914
The US Congress establishes the Federal Trade Commission (FTC) for the purpose of preventing unfair methods of competition in commerce.

1906
The US Congress passes the Federal Food and Drugs Act, which is the first legislation to protect consumers from misbranded or harmful foods, drugs, medicines, and liquors.

1902
Kellogg cereals magnate Frank J. Kellogg introduces Rengo, which he says is the first drug that can reduce fat. When the drug is found to disrupt heart rhythm and weaken the heart muscle, it is withdrawn from the market.

1997

Mayo Clinic physician Heidi Connelly publishes an article in the *New England Journal of Medicine* about heart valve abnormalities among twenty-four women who were taking the combination of fenfluramine and phentermine. After other similar reports surface, fenfluramine and a hybrid drug called Redux are withdrawn from the market by the FDA.

2011

US Senator Dick Durbin introduces the Dietary Supplement Labeling Act, a bill that is intended to improve the safety of dietary supplements by requiring manufacturers to register them with the FDA.

2010

A clinical trial that involves nearly ten thousand overweight or obese people finds that the diet pill Meridia increases the risks of heart attacks and strokes while not being an effective weight-loss drug.

1990

2000

2010

1994

With Congress's passage of the Dietary Supplement Health and Education Act, dietary supplements are defined as foods rather than drugs, which removes them from FDA oversight.

2012

After thirteen years of no new weight-loss drugs being released, the FDA approves two new drugs: Belviq and Qsymia.

2004

The Food and Drug Administration bans the stimulant ephedra from being an ingredient in any supplements or drugs (including those for weight loss) sold in the United States.

2013

A study by the market research firm Marketdata finds that total sales of all diet- and weight-loss-related products totaled $61.56 billion in 2012, with prescription diet drugs representing only one-half percent of the total amount.

1992

University of Rochester pharmacologist Michael Weintraub publishes an article about an effective weight-loss regimen that combines the drugs fenfluramine and phentermine, which comes to be known as fen-phen. Popularity of the combination drug skyrockets.

Related Organizations

Academy of Nutrition and Dietetics

120 S. Riverside Plaza, Suite 2000
Chicago, IL 60606-6995
phone: (312) 899-0040; toll-free: (800) 877-1600
website: www.eatright.org

Formerly the American Dietetic Association, the Academy of Nutrition and Dietetics seeks to improve Americans' health and advance the profession of dietetics through research, education, and advocacy. Its website search engine produces articles about weight loss and diet drugs.

Alliance for Natural Health

6931 Arlington Rd., Suite 304
Bethesda, MD 20814
phone: (800) 230-2762 • fax: (202) 315-5837
website: www.anh-usa.org

The Alliance for Natural Health is an advocacy organization that promotes a healthy diet and lifestyle and favors alternative medicine over drugs, surgery, and other conventional techniques. Its website links to numerous publications about diet drugs and dietary supplements.

Federal Trade Commission (FTC)

600 Pennsylvania Ave. NW
Washington, DC 20580
phone: (202) 326-2222; toll-free: (877) 382-4357
website: www.ftc.gov

The FTC is charged with protecting American consumers from fraud, deception, and unfair business practices. Its website search engine produces a number of articles about weight-loss products and supplements.

Mayo Clinic

200 First St. SW
Rochester, MN 55905
phone: (507) 284-2511
website: www.mayoclinic.com

The Mayo Clinic is a world-renowned medical facility that is dedicated to patient care, education, and research. Its website search engine produces many informative articles about over-the-counter and prescription weight-loss drugs and supplements.

National Center for Complementary and Alternative Medicine (NCCAM)

9000 Rockville Pike
Bethesda, MD 20892
phone: (888) 644-6226
website: http://nccam.nih.gov

Through scientific research, the NCCAM investigates the usefulness and safety of complementary and alternative medical treatments in improving health and health care. Its website search engine produces numerous articles related to weight loss, drugs, and supplements.

National Institute of Diabetes and Digestive and Kidney Diseases (NIDDK)

Bldg. 31, Room 9A06, MSC 2560
31 Center Dr., MSC 2560
Bethesda, MD 20892-2560
phone: (301) 496-3583
e-mail: nddic@info.niddk.nih.gov
website: http://digestive.niddk.nih.gov

An agency of the National Institutes of Health, the NIDDK conducts and supports medical research and research training to improve the health and quality of life of people suffering from diabetes and digestive and kidney diseases. Its website links to the National Digestive Diseases Information Clearinghouse, which is its information dissemination service.

Obesity Action Coalition

4511 North Himes Ave., Suite 250
Tampa, FL 33614
phone: (813) 872-7835 • fax (813) 873-7838
e-mail: info@obesityaction.org • website: obesityaction.org

The Obesity Action Coalition seeks to raise awareness of obesity, ensure access to safe and effective treatment options, and eradicate the negative bias and stigma associated with obesity. Its website offers educational resources, information about treating obesity, and a search engine that produces a collection of articles about weight-loss techniques, including medications.

Office of Dietary Supplements

National Institutes of Health
6100 Executive Blvd., Room 3B01, MSC 7517
Bethesda, MD 20892-7517
phone: (301) 435-2920 • toll free: (800) 717-3117
fax: (301) 480-1845
e-mail: ods@nih.gov • website: http://ods.od.nih.gov

The Office of Dietary Supplements seeks to strengthen knowledge and understanding of dietary supplements through research and public education. Its website offers news releases, fact sheets, consumer updates, and a search engine that produces numerous articles about supplements, including those that are designed to help with weight loss.

US Food and Drug Administration (FDA)

10903 New Hampshire Ave.
Silver Spring, MD 20993-0022
phone: (888) 463-6332
website: www.fda.gov

The FDA is responsible for protecting the public health by assuring the safety and effectiveness of America's food supply, human and veterinary drugs, and other products. A number of articles and podcasts about diet drugs can be accessed through the agency's website.

Yale University Rudd Center for Food Policy & Obesity

Rudd Center for Food Policy & Obesity
Yale University
309 Edwards St.
New Haven, CT 06511
phone: (203) 432-6700 • fax: (203) 432-9674
e-mail: rudd.center@yale.edu • website: www.yaleruddcenter.org

The Rudd Center for Food Policy & Obesity is a nonprofit research and public policy organization that seeks to improve the world's diet, prevent obesity, and reduce weight stigma. Its website offers a wide variety of information about obesity-related issues, including some articles about diet drugs.

For Further Research

Books

Vincent Bellonzi, *Health Recklessly Abandoned: Take Back Control of Your Own Health and Live the Life You Deserve*. Garden City, NY: Morgan James, 2013.

Elaine A. Moore, *The Amphetamine Debate: The Use of Adderall, Ritalin and Related Drugs for Behavior Modification, Neuroenhancement and Anti-Aging Purposes*. Jefferson, NC: McFarland, 2011.

Pamela A. Popper and Glen Merzer, *Food Over Medicine: The Conversation That Could Save Your Life*. Dallas, TX: BenBella, 2013.

Alex Rogers, *Weight Loss and Fat Burning: Suckers, Scams, Lies, Fad Diets, Bogus Products, and How Not to Become a Victim of the Weight-Loss Industry and How to Start Losing Fat Now!* Brick, NJ: Alex Rogers, 2012.

Periodicals

Alex Ballingall, "New Diet Features a Lick of Lizard Spit: Rats Fed a Substance Found in Gila Monster Saliva Crave Less Food," *Maclean's*, vol. 125, no. 2, June 4, 2012.

Berkeley Wellness, "Diet Drugs: Déjà Vu All Over Again?," June 2013.

Andrea Davis, "Obesity Drugs: Fat-Fighting Drugs No Silver Bullet for Beating Obesity," *Employee Benefit News*, March 1, 2013.

Katie Drummond, "Diet-Drug Underground," *New York*, February 26, 2012.

Economist, "Slim Pickings: Treating Obesity," December 15, 2012.

Melanie Haiken, "5 Deadliest Diet Trends: Pills That Really Can Kill," *Forbes*, April 19, 2012.

Nanci Hellmich, "Diet Drugs Have Had a Rocky History," *USA Today*, June 27, 2012.

Andrew Pollack, "Side Effects of Diet Pill Still Concern Regulators," *New York Times*, February 17, 2012.

Sophie Quinton, "FDA, FTC Crack Down on Illegal Weight-Loss Products," *National Journal*, December 6, 2011.

Kate Ryan, "Weight Loss Products: Do They Improve Health?," *Women's Health Activist*, May 2011.

Judy Stone, "A Glut of Obesity Drugs?," *Scientific American*, July 2, 2012.

USA Today, "When Less Food Means More Weight," September 2012.

Vogue, "The Quick Fix," January 2013.

Internet Sources

Kathleen Doheny, "The Real Dangers of Weight-Loss Drugs," *Consumers Digest*, May 2011. www.consumersdigest.com/health/the-real-dangers-of-weight-loss-drugs.

Food and Drug Administration, "6 Tip-Offs to Rip-Offs: Don't Fall for Health Fraud Scams," March 2013. www.fda.gov/downloads/For Consumers/ConsumerUpdates/UCM342124.pdf.

National Institute of Diabetes and Digestive and Kidney Diseases, "Prescription Medications for the Treatment of Obesity," December 2010. http://win.niddk.nih.gov/publications/prescription.htm.

Kent Sepkowitz, "Why New Diet Drugs, Belviq and Qsymia, Are Just in Time," *Daily Beast*, July 19, 2012. www.thedailybeast.com/articles/2012/07/19/new-diet-drugs-get-green-light-just-as-u-s-obesity-epidemic-deepens.html.

Alexandra Sifferlin, "For Successful Weight Loss, Forget Fad Diets and Pills," *Time*, April 10, 2012. http://healthland.time.com/2012/04/10/for-successful-weight-loss-forget-fad-diets-and-pills.

Felicia Stoler, "The Skinny on FDA Regulation of Dietary Supplements," Fox News, March 23, 2012. www.foxnews.com/health/2012/03/23/skinny-on-fda-regulation-dietary-supplements.

Bob Trebilcock, "If Your Diet Drug Works . . . It's Bad for You," *Prevention*, November 2011. www.prevention.com/mind-body/natural-remedies/diet-pill-dangers-truth-behind-weight-loss-supplements.

Katie Valentine, "Biggest Loser Trainers Publicly Promote Diet and Exercise, Quietly Endorse Unproven Weight Loss Pills," *Think Progress* (blog), March 17, 2013. http://thinkprogress.org/health/2013/03/17/1715601/biggest-loser-trainers-diet-pills.

Source Notes

Overview

1. Quoted in Nanci Hellmich, "New Diet Drug Helps Patients Lose About 10% of Weight," *USA Today*, July 18, 2012. http://usatoday30.usatoday.com.
2. Sandra Adamson Fryhofer, "Lorcaserin: The Second Weight-Loss Contender," Medscape Today, September 7, 2012. www.medscape.com.
3. Kelly Brownell, in "Pounding Away at America's Obesity Epidemic," NPR, May 14, 2012. www.npr.org.
4. Mayo Clinic, "Over-the-Counter Weight-Loss Pills: Do They Work?," February 11, 2012. www.mayoclinic.com.
5. NIDDK, "Prescription Medications for the Treatment of Obesity," November 16, 2012. http://win.niddk.nih.gov.
6. Kathleen Donnelly, "Diet Pills: A Dubious History of Problems," MSN Healthy Living. Accessed June 10, 2013. http://healthyliving.msn.com.
7. FDAImports.com, "Drugs," 2013. www.fdaimports.com.
8. Susan Thaul, *How FDA Approves Drugs and Regulates Their Safety and Effectiveness*, Congressional Research Service, June 25, 2012. www.fas.org.
9. US Food and Drug Administration, "Beware of Fraudulent Weight-Loss 'Dietary Supplements'—They Can Kill You!," April 18, 2013. www.fda.gov. FDA Advisor.
10. Yoni Freedhoff and Arya M. Sharma, "'Lose 40 Pounds in 4 Weeks': Regulating Commercial Weight Loss Programs," *Canadian Medical Association Journal*, February 17, 2009. www.cmaj.ca.
11. Quoted in Courtney Hutchison, "Snooki Pushes Zantrex-3 Diet Pill, Docs Disapprove," ABC News, September 28, 2011. http://abcnews.go.com.
12. Stephan Guyenet, "Qsymia (formerly Qnexa), the Latest Obesity Drug," *Whole Health Source* (blog), March 17, 2012. http://wholehealthsource.blogspot.com.
13. Quoted in Melissa Dahl, "Diet Pill's Icky Side Effects Keep Users Honest," NBC News, July 6, 2007. www.nbcnews.com.
14. Berkeley Wellness, "Diet Drugs: Déjà Vu All Over Again?," June 4, 2013, p. 6.

What Are Diet Drugs?

15. Quoted in Liz Brody, "Are Two Diet Pills Better than One?," *USA Today*, March 8, 2011. www.today.com.
16. Melinda Beck, "New Diet Pills Offer Option to Off-Label Obesity Drugs," *Wall Street Journal*, July 30, 2012. http://online.wsj.com.
17. Beck, "New Diet Pills Offer Option to Off-Label Obesity Drugs."
18. Quoted in Brody, "Are Two Diet Pills Better than One?"
19. Quoted in Joan Raymond, "Antidepressants and Other 'New' Diet Pills: Do They Work, and Are They Safe?" *Health*, February 22, 2008. www.health.com.
20. Quoted in Raymond, "Antidepressants and Other 'New' Diet Pills."
21. Quoted in Brody, "Are Two Diet Pills Better than One?"
22. Alicia Mundy, *Dispensing with the Truth: The Victims, the Drug Companies, and the Dramatic Story Behind the Battle Over Fen-Phen*. New York: St. Martin's, 2001. http://pubs.acs.org.

23. Quoted in Lawrence Bachorik, "FDA Announces Withdrawal Fenfluramine and Dexfenfluramine (Fen-Phen)," US Food and Drug Administration, September 15, 1997. www.fda.gov.
24. Quoted in Beck, "New Diet Pills Offer Option to Off-Label Obesity Drugs."
25. Quoted in John Bowersox, "NIAAA Researchers Advance Potential Obesity Treatment," National Institute on Alcohol Abuse and Alcoholism, August 3, 2012. www.niaaa.nih .gov.

How Effective Are Diet Drugs?

26. Quoted in Elisa Lipsky-Karasz, "From a Size 14 to a Size 4," *Harper's Bazaar*, May 2010. www.harpersbazaar.com.
27. Quoted in Lipsky-Karasz, "From a Size 14 to a Size 4."
28. Quoted in Kathleen Doheny, "The Real Dangers of Weight-Loss Drugs," *Consumers Digest*, May 2011. www.consumersdigest.com.
29. Quoted in Lipsky-Karasz, "From a Size 14 to a Size 4."
30. Quoted in Rachael Rettner, "Drug Combo Shows Promise for Obesity Treatment," *MyHealthNewsDaily*, April 11, 2011. www.myhealthnewsdaily.com.
31. Meredith C. Fiddler et al., "A One-Year Randomized Trial of Lorcaserin for Weight Loss in Obese and Overweight Adults: The BLOSSOM Trial," *Journal of Clinical Endocrinology & Metabolism*, October 2011. http://jcem.endojournals.org.
32. Steven Novella, "Weight Loss Supplements Don't Work," *NeuroLogica blog*, March 8, 2012. http://theness.com.
33. Quoted in Katie Valentine, "Biggest Loser Trainers Publicly Promote Diet and Exercise, Quietly Endorse Unproven Weight Loss Pills," *ThinkProgress Health* (blog), March 17, 2013. http://thinkprogress.org.
34. Quoted in Jennipher Walters, "Are Weight-Loss Supplements Effective? Study Says Most Aren't," *Shape*, March 19, 2012. www.shape.com.
35. Quoted in Walters, "Are Weight-Loss Supplements Effective?"
36. Quoted in Tim Boyer, "Coffee Bean Diet Results in Fast Weight Loss Announced at American Chemical Society," *EmaxHealth*, March 27, 2012. www.emaxhealth.com.

What Are the Health Risks of Diet Drugs?

37. Quoted in Chris Brooke, "Banned Slimming Drug Kills Medical Student: Coroner Attacks Online Dealers Who Target the Vulnerable," *Daily Mail*, April 22, 2013. www .dailymail.co.uk.
38. Quoted in Brooke, "Banned Slimming Drug Kills Medical Student."
39. Pieter A. Cohen, "American Roulette—Contaminated Dietary Supplements," *New England Journal of Medicine*, October 15, 2009. www.nejm.org.
40. Quoted in US Food and Drug Administration, "Beware of Fraudulent Weight-Loss 'Dietary Supplements,'" March 15, 2011. www.fda.gov.
41. Quoted in Natasha Singer, "F.D.A. Finds 'Natural Diet Pills' Laced with Drugs," *New York Times*, February 9, 2009. www.nytimes.com.
42. Quoted in *Consumer Reports*, "Weight-Loss Drugs: Alli and Xenical (Orlistat)," August 2009. www.consumerreports.org.
43. Quoted in *Science Daily*, "Most Popular Weight-Loss Drug Strongly Alters Other Drug Therapies, Study Suggests," December 10, 2012. www.sciencedaily.com.
44. Quoted in *Science Daily*, "Most Popular Weight-Loss Drug Strongly Alters Other Drug Therapies, Study Suggests."

45. US Department of Health and Human Services, "Why Is Ephedra Banned by the FDA?," November 7, 2012. http://answers.hhs.gov.

46. Quoted in Antonia Hoyle, "Michelle Thought Diet Pills Could Help Her Drop a Dress Size. Now She's Got Just Ten Years to Live," *Daily Mail*, September 19, 2012. www .dailymail.co.uk.

47. Quoted in Hoyle, "Michelle Thought Diet Pills Could Help Her Drop a Dress Size."

48. Quoted in Hoyle, "Michelle Thought Diet Pills Could Help Her Drop a Dress Size."

How Big a Problem Is Diet-Drug Fraud?

49. Quoted in Federal Trade Commission, "Fake News," April 2011. www.ftc.gov.

50. Quoted in Federal Trade Commission, "Fake News."

51. Quoted in Federal Trade Commission, "FTC Seeks to Halt 10 Operators of Fake News Sites from Making Deceptive Claims About Acai Berry Weight Loss Products," April 2011. www.consumer.ftc.gov.

52. Federal Trade Commission, "Fake News Sites Promote Acai Supplements," July 2012. www.consumer.ftc.gov.

53. Federal Trade Commission, "FTC Seeks to Halt 10 Operators of Fake News Sites from Making Deceptive Claims About Acai Berry Weight Loss Products."

54. Quoted in Kevin Hunt, "Guilford Man's $25 Million Weight-Loss Scam: Why People Fell for It," *Hartford (CT) Courant*, January 28, 2012. http://articles.courant.com.

55. Quoted in Hunt, "Guilford Man's $25 Million Weight-Loss Scam."

56. Quoted in Hunt, "Guilford Man's $25 Million Weight-Loss Scam."

57. Quoted in Hunt, "Guilford Man's $25 Million Weight-Loss Scam."

58. Food and Drug Administration, "6 Tip-Offs to Rip-Offs: Don't Fall for Health Fraud Scams," March 2013. www.fda.gov.

59. Federal Trade Commission, *Consumer Fraud in the United States, 2011: The Third FTC Survey*, April 2013. www.ftc.gov.

60. Novella, "Weight Loss Supplements Don't Work."

61. Quoted in *HealthDay*, "FDA Targets Homeopathic Weight Loss Products," December 6, 2011. http://consumer.healthday.com.

62. Quoted in *HealthDay*, "FDA Targets Homeopathic Weight Loss Products."

List of Illustrations

Index

About the Author

Peggy J. Parks holds a bachelor of science degree from Aquinas College in Grand Rapids, Michigan, where she graduated magna cum laude. An author who has written more than a hundred educational books for children and young adults, Parks lives in Muskegon, Michigan, a town that she says inspires her writing because of its location on the shores of Lake Michigan.